LONGEVITY SECRETS

The Ultimate Guide to Aging Gracefully and Lifelong Wellness

MAXWELL MASON

TABLE OF CONTENTS

Introduction   7

CHAPTER 1   11
1.1 Deciphering the Longevity Code: Telomeres and
Aging   14
1.2 The Impact of Chronic Inflammation on Aging   15
1.3 Autophagy: The Body's Natural Detoxifying
Process   19

2. THE MIND'S INFLUENCE ON LONGEVITY   23
2.1 Cultivating a Growth Mindset for Ageless
Living   23
2.2 The Link Between Emotional Health and
Longevity   26
2.3 Overcoming Age-Related Mental Health
Challenges   29
2.4 Harnessing the Power of Resilience and
Adaptability   31

3. NOURISHING LONGEVITY: THE POWER
OF DIET   35
3.1 The Longevity Diet: Foods That Fight Aging   35
3.2 Superfoods for Superior Health: Beyond
the Hype   39
3.3 Navigating Dietary Supplements for Aging
Adults   41
3.4 Intermittent Fasting and Circadian Rhythms   44

4. MOVEMENT AS MEDICINE   47
4.1 Tailoring Your Exercise Regimen to Your Age   47
4.2 The Science of Strength Training for Seniors   50
4.3 Low-Impact Workouts: Effective Options for
Every Fitness Level   52
4.4 The Role of Flexibility and Balance in Aging
Gracefully   56

5. BIOHACKING YOUR WAY TO OPTIMAL
HEALTH   59
    5.1 Red-Light Therapy: Skin Health and Beyond   59
    5.2 The Benefits of Cold Exposure: Myth vs.
Reality   63
    5.3 Elevating Health with Hydrogen Water   66
    5.4 Grounding: Connecting with the Earth's Energy   68

6. NOURISHING LONGEVITY FROM THE
WORLD'S BLUE ZONES   71
    6.1 Dietary Secrets from the Blue Zones   71
    6.2 Community and Social Connections: Learning
from Okinawa   73
    6.3 Stress Management Techniques from the
World's Oldest People   76
    6.4 Physical Activity as a Way of Life in Longevity
Cultures   79

7. MINDFULNESS AND MEDITATION: PATHWAYS
TO LONGEVITY   83
    7.1 The Science of Meditation and Mindfulness in
Longevity   83
    7.2 Yoga and Tai Chi: Physical Benefits and Beyond   86
    7.3 Biofeedback and Neurofeedback for Emotional
Regulation   88
    7.4 The Healing Power of Breathwork   90

8. DIGITAL HARMONY: RECLAIMING PRESENCE
IN THE AGE OF DISTRACTION   95
    8.1 Digital Detoxing: Balancing Technology in
Your Life   95
    8.2 The Impact of Environmental Toxins on Health   98
    8.3 Strategies for Managing Information Overload   100
    8.4 Sleep Hygiene for the 21st Century   102

9. NURTURING THE SELF: A BLUEPRINT FOR
PERSONALIZED WELLNESS   107
    9.1 Assessing Your Health and Wellness Goals   107
    9.2 Integrating Biohacks into Your Daily Routine   110
    9.3 Setting Realistic, Achievable Health Milestones   112
    9.4 Tracking Progress: Tools and Technologies   114

10. CULTIVATING COLLECTIVE WELLNESS: A
SYMPHONY OF SUPPORT 119
 10.1 Building a Supportive Wellness Community 119
 10.2 The Benefits of Group Exercise and Social
 Activities 121
 10.3 Volunteering: Giving Back for Your Health 124
 10.4 Nurturing Relationships for Mental and
 Emotional Health 126

11. SOOTHING THE SENSES: NATURE'S BALM FOR
JOINT HEALTH 131
 11.1 Natural Approaches to Managing Joint Pain
 and Arthritis 131
 11.2 Cognitive Health: Preventing Memory Loss
 and Dementia 134
 11.3 Heart Health: Combating the #1 Killer with
 Lifestyle Changes 136
 11.4 Diabetes Prevention and Management Through
 Lifestyle 139

12. EMBRACING THE HORIZON: THE VANGUARD
OF LONGEVITY SCIENCE 143
 12.2 The Next Generation of Biohacks: What's on
 the Horizon 146
 12.3 The Role of Personalized Medicine in Wellness 148
 12.4 Staying Ahead: Continuous Learning for
 Lifelong Health 150

Conclusion 155
References 159

INTRODUCTION

There's a timeless adage that compares the human body to a sophisticated machine—a marvel of nature that thrives on balance, care, and continuous renewal. Just as the most advanced machines require regular upkeep and occasional enhancements to function at their peak, so too does our biological machinery. This book is an invitation to explore the myriad ways we can tune, refine, and sometimes, fundamentally upgrade our systems using the dual lenses of cutting-edge biohacks and age-old wisdom.

Though not significant, my name represents every individual who has allowed life's incessant demands to overshadow their well-being. I found myself navigating through a maze of health challenges, including prediabetes and ankylosing spondylitis, all while watching my wife fight for her life in the ICU, a stark wake-up call that shifted my priorities towards health and longevity. These personal trials ignited an emotional quest to not only reclaim my health but to understand how I could sustain it through the decades ahead.

This book is born out of a deep desire to share the treasures unearthed on this journey. It's crafted for you—the modern individual who stands at the crossroads of advancing age and the aspiration for a life brimming with energy, purpose, and health. Whether you're in your prime years, wondering how to maintain your vigor, or you've noticed the subtle signs of aging and seek to slow its tide, this guide is your companion.

The profound connection between mind and body is at the heart of our exploration—a relationship so intricate that our mental and emotional states can profoundly influence our physical health. We'll delve into stress management techniques, the importance of restorative sleep, and ways to nurture our mental and emotional landscapes, all underpinned by the philosophy that true wellness encompasses the whole self.

I'm excited to introduce you to a world where biohacking meets traditional health practices, where insights from experts like Gary Brecka illuminate our path. We'll investigate the benefits of red-light therapy, the grounding effects of connecting with the Earth, and the rejuvenating properties of hydrogen water, among other innovations. These topics don't just represent chapters in a book; they are keys to unlocking a more vibrant, resilient you.

You, the reader, are the reason this book exists. Whether you're an adult stepping into the second act of your life or a senior seeking to invigorate your golden years, this guide is tailored for you. It's structured to walk you through the foundational principles of longevity, actionable strategies for wellness, and into the horizon of future research and practices.

Let this book be your motivation to approach your wellness journey with curiosity and dedication. The chapters that follow are more than just pages of information; they are stepping stones to a fuller, richer life. I invite you not just to read but to engage deeply with the exercises, examples, and recommendations within these pages.

Your journey to longevity and wellness starts now. Let's turn the page together and unlock the secrets to a life of vitality and fulfillment.

CHAPTER ONE

In the realm of longevity, a familiar anecdote often surfaces about the centenarians of Okinawa who seemingly bypass the conventional effects of aging, leading lives marked by vitality and health well into their final decades. This phenomenon prompts a compelling question: Are these remarkable lifespans a courtesy of their genetic lottery, or are they the cumulative result of lifestyle choices sculpted over a lifetime? The answer lies in the intricate dance between our genetic blueprint and the daily decisions we make—a relationship that profoundly influences our journey toward a long, healthy life.

The Role of Genetics vs. Lifestyle in Longevity

Genetic Predisposition and Its Impact

Our genetic makeup undoubtedly sets the stage for our health outcomes. It's akin to inheriting a map that outlines the potential paths our health might take. Specific genes, for instance, are directly linked to a longer lifespan, offering some individuals a head start in the race toward longevity. Research in the field of genomics has shed light on markers such as the FOXO3 gene associated with increased lifespan across diverse populations. However, it's critical to understand that our genes are not our destiny. They provide a framework within which a vast array of possibilities exists, heavily influenced by our environment and behavior.

The Power of Lifestyle Modifications

Lifestyle modifications play a pivotal role within this space of possibility. The burgeoning field of epigenetics offers a fascinating insight into how our environment and choices can modify the expression of our genes without altering the DNA sequence itself. For example, regular physical activity and a diet rich in antioxidants can activate pathways that enhance DNA repair and cellular maintenance, effectively decelerating the aging process. This concept is not merely theoretical; a study published in the journal *Nature* demonstrated how lifestyle interventions could significantly extend the lifespan of mice by modifying the activity of age-related genes. The implications for human health are profound, suggesting that our daily habits wield the power to influence our genetic expression in favor of longevity.

Nature vs. Nurture Debate in Longevity

The intersection of genetics and lifestyle in determining our healthspan revitalizes the age-old nature versus nurture debate. In the context of longevity, it becomes increasingly clear that neither genetics nor lifestyle singularly dictates our fate. Instead, the interplay between the two sets the course of our health trajectory. Consider the Mediterranean diet, celebrated for its cardiovascular benefits. While individuals in the Mediterranean region enjoy a genetic predisposition to heart health, their adherence to a diet low in saturated fats and high in fruits, vegetables, and whole grains amplifies this genetic advantage. Thus, the secret to a long, vibrant life does not rest solely in our genetic code but also in the lifestyle choices we make every day.

Personalizing Wellness Strategies

The realization that lifestyle can influence genetic expression underscores the importance of personalizing wellness strategies. In an era where genetic testing is increasingly accessible, individuals have the unique opportunity to tailor their lifestyle interventions based on their genetic predispositions. For instance, someone with a genetic variant that affects vitamin D metabolism may benefit from tailored dietary adjustments to optimize their vitamin D levels. This personalized approach extends beyond nutrition into physical activity, stress management, and sleep habits, allowing for a customized blueprint for longevity.

Taking this personalized path requires a deep understanding of one's unique genetic makeup and the lifestyle factors that can mitigate or exacerbate genetic risks. It's akin to navigating a complex terrain with a compass pointing to health optimization. By making informed choices about our diet, exercise, and other lifestyle factors, we can nudge our genetic predispositions toward a longer, healthier life.

In this pursuit of longevity, the fusion of genetic understanding and lifestyle adaptation emerges as a powerful strategy. It offers a roadmap for navigating the complexities of aging, empowering us with the knowledge and tools needed to sculpt our health destiny. With each lifestyle choice, we can influence our genetic expression, unlocking the potential for a life that spans decades and is rich in vitality and wellness.

1.1 DECIPHERING THE LONGEVITY CODE: TELOMERES AND AGING

At the cellular level, aging manifests as a slow, inevitable march toward dysfunction, with telomeres standing as vigilant guardians at the chromosomal frontiers. These structures, composed of repetitive nucleotide sequences, cap the ends of chromosomes, safeguarding them from deterioration or fusion with neighboring chromosomes. Yet, with each cellular division, telomeres undergo a reduction in length, a process subtly orchestrated in the backdrop of our biological aging narrative. This gradual shortening is a biomarker of cellular age, suggesting a direct correlation between telomere length and the aging process.

The influence of lifestyle on the integrity of these chromosomal protectors reveals a compelling facet of the aging puzzle. For instance, a diet rich in antioxidants acts as a bulwark against oxidative stress, a known accelerant of telomere shortening. Omega-3 fatty acids found abundantly in fish, have been observed to foster telomere maintenance, offering a dietary angle to the quest for elongated healthspan. Beyond nutrition, stress management emerges as a pivotal factor in telomere preservation. Chronic stress, with its insidious release of cortisol, has been implicated in the accelerated erosion of telomere length, positioning relaxation, and mindfulness practices as essential tools in the longevity toolkit. Moreover, by mitigating stress and enhancing antioxidant defenses, physical activity stands as a robust ally in the defense against premature telomere attrition.

Telomerase, the enzyme responsible for adding nucleotide sequences to telomeres, thus extending their length and potentially the lifespan of cells, becomes a beacon of hope in the quest for extended youthfulness. Telomerase activation through natural means—such as specific lifestyle interventions—presents a compelling avenue for longevity research. While direct telomerase stimulation remains a complex challenge, emerging evidence suggests that holistic health practices may indirectly bolster its activity, offering a glimpse into potential strategies for decelerating the aging process.

The empirical landscape teems with studies that underscore the relationship between telomere length and longevity practices. Research has illuminated the positive impact of meditation on telomere maintenance, with practitioners exhibiting less telomere shortening compared to non-meditators, a testament to the power of stress reduction in cellular aging. Similarly, investigations into the effects of aerobic exercise have revealed its capacity to preserve telomere length, highlighting physical activity's role in curtailing the biological markers of aging. These findings, among others, stitch together a narrative where lifestyle choices become critical determinants of cellular aging, offering a blueprint for interventions to extend health span.

In this exploration of telomeres and their intricate role in the aging process, we encounter a crossroads where biology meets lifestyle, where the microscopic and the macroscopic intertwine in the dance of aging. The evidence suggests that through mindful attention to diet, stress, and physical well-being, we possess the capacity to influence our cellular destiny, perhaps unlocking the secrets to a longer, healthier life.

1.2 THE IMPACT OF CHRONIC INFLAMMATION ON AGING

At the cellular level, the body's response to injury or threat—namely, inflammation—serves as a protective mechanism designed to safeguard the organism from external invaders and initiate the healing process. Yet, when this response lingers, failing to dissipate after the danger has been neutralized, it morphs into a slow-burning fire known as chronic inflammation. This persistent state, marked by the constant production of inflammatory cytokines, subtly undermines our physiological integrity, contributing to the gradual erosion of cellular function that characterizes aging.

The sources of inflammation are as varied as they are pervasive, spanning from dietary indiscretions to environmental toxins. Processed foods, rich in refined sugars and trans fats, act as kindling, fueling the inflammatory response, while sedentary lifestyles further exacerbate this condition, allowing inflammation to simmer unchecked. Environmental pollutants, including particulate matter from air pollution and synthetic chemicals in household products, serve as additional catalysts, igniting inflammatory pathways within the body. Even psychological stress, through the insidious release of cortisol, can fan the flames of inflammation, illustrating the complex interplay between the mind and physiological processes.

Navigating the multifaceted landscape of chronic inflammation requires a nuanced, strategic approach emphasizing deliberate lifestyle adjustments to quell the persistent inflammatory response. Central to these adjustments is the transformative power of diet, focusing on whole, nutrient-dense foods that serve as natural anti-inflammatories. Embarking on a dietary journey rich in leafy greens, such as spinach and kale, vibrant berries packed with antioxidants, and omega-3-rich fatty fish like salmon and mackerel offers a robust defense against inflammation. These foods, celebrated for their high antioxidant and phytonutrient content, not only counteract the oxidative stress underlying inflammation but also nurture the body's intrinsic healing mechanisms. Complementing dietary modifications and integrating regular, consistent physical activity into one's daily regimen is a pivotal strategy for combating chronic inflammation. Exercise, particularly when it encompasses moderate-intensity activities like brisk walking, cycling, or swimming, initiates a cascade of biochemical reactions that elevate mood, enhance cardiovascular health, and significantly reduce inflammatory markers. This activity-induced reduction in inflammation functions akin to a soothing balm, tempering the internal inflammatory milieu and fostering an environment conducive to cellular repair and rejuvenation. Together, these anti-inflammatory lifestyle adjustments forge a pathway to mitigating the insidious effects of chronic inflammation, spotlighting the critical role of diet and exercise in preserving cellular integrity and promoting a state of enduring vitality and wellness.

When judiciously incorporated, supplementation is a powerful ally in the fight against chronic inflammation. Among the pantheon of natural supplements, curcumin — the bioactive compound found in turmeric — stands out for its remarkable anti-inflammatory prowess. Scientific research underscores curcumin's ability to inhibit critical enzymes and cytokines involved in the inflammatory process, offering a natural, complementary strategy for dampening inflammation. Its effectiveness, however, is contingent upon adequate absorption, a challenge that can be addressed by combining curcumin with piperine, a compound in black pepper known to enhance bioavailability. Equally significant in the anti-inflammatory arsenal are omega-3 fatty acids, hailed for their capacity to modulate the body's inflammatory response. These essential fats, particularly EPA (eicosapentaenoic acid) and DHA (docosahexaenoic acid), have been extensively studied for their role in reducing the production of inflammatory eicosanoids and cytokines. Available through both diets — in fatty fish like salmon, mackerel, and sardines — and high-quality supplements, omega-3s contribute to a holistic anti-inflammatory regimen, supporting cardiovascular health, cognitive function, and overall well-being. These supplements should be incorporated with an understanding of their synergistic potential and the nuances of individual health profiles, ensuring that they complement dietary and lifestyle strategies to mitigate inflammation and promote longevity.

Measuring and monitoring inflammation necessitates a grasp of the biomarkers that signal its presence. High-sensitivity C-reactive protein (hs-CRP) emerges as a critical indicator, providing insight into systemic inflammation with a simple blood test. Similarly, levels of interleukin-6 and tumor necrosis factor-alpha offer a window into the body's inflammatory state, allowing for targeted interventions. Monitoring these markers, particularly in individuals with known risk factors for chronic diseases, can guide lifestyle modifications, enabling a tailored approach to mitigate inflammation.

This narrative profoundly resonates with me due to a personal health revelation at 44, when routine blood tests revealed elevated levels of C-reactive protein—a key marker indicating inflammation within my body. Shortly after that, I was diagnosed with ankylosing spondylitis, a type of arthritis that primarily affects the spine, leading to severe, chronic pain and discomfort. The prescribed course of action was a bi-weekly regimen of biologic infusion treatments, a routine that remains a part of my life today. Initially, one might anticipate that such a diagnosis would lead to an immediate, comprehensive overhaul of one's health strategy, prompting a thorough investigation into the efficacy of biologic treatments alongside supplementary lifestyle changes to combat the condition. However, I found myself trapped by a common misconception: the belief that the entirety of my treatment and health management should be left in the hands of healthcare professionals, with no need for personal intervention or adjustment. As a result, for nearly a decade, I overlooked the critical importance of diet modification, the introduction of targeted supplements, and the incorporation of regular, meaningful exercise into my daily routine. My focus remained steadfastly on my career, to the detriment of my health. This period of inaction persisted until a significant health crisis with my wife served as a stark wake-up call, highlighting the urgent need for proactive personal health management. Reflecting on this journey, it's evident that chronic inflammation is not merely a symptom to be treated in isolation but a crucial factor in the aging process that can insidiously undermine our vitality and wellness from within. It's a stark reminder of the necessity to actively engage in our health strategy actively, understanding and addressing the myriad sources of chronic inflammation. Through a committed approach to dietary choices, regular physical activity, and appropriate supplementation, we can safeguard our cellular integrity, enhancing our overall health and longevity. This personal experience underlines the profound impact that informed, deliberate health decisions can have on our quality of life, reinforcing the message that taking control of one's health is not just beneficial but essential for a vibrant, fulfilling future.

1.3 AUTOPHAGY: THE BODY'S NATURAL DETOXIFYING PROCESS

In the intricate ballet of cellular function, autophagy plays a pivotal role, akin to an unseen custodian tirelessly working to maintain cleanliness and order within. This self-eating mechanism, a term derived from the Greek words for "self" and "eating," refers to the process by which cells deconstruct and recycle their own components. This continual cycle of renewal is fundamental to cellular health and, by extension, the organism's vitality. Within this self-regulatory system, damaged organelles, misfolded proteins, and other cellular debris are encapsulated in vesicles known as autophagosomes, which subsequently fuse with lysosomes to degrade the encapsulated material, thereby sustaining cellular homeostasis and promoting longevity.

Activating or enhancing autophagy through lifestyle choices is a powerful adjunct to the body's natural detoxifying processes. Periods of fasting initiate a survival mechanism within cells, triggering autophagy to conserve energy and generate vital nutrients from within. This process is not merely a byproduct of energy conservation but a deliberate, adaptive response honed through millennia of evolutionary pressures, enabling organisms to thrive during times of scarcity. Similarly, physical exercise, by placing transient stress on the body, activates a compensatory response that includes the upregulation of autophagy, thus contributing to improved cellular function and resistance to stressors.

Moreover, the inclusion of specific nutrients in the diet can modulate autophagy pathways. Compounds such as spermidine, found in aged cheese, mushrooms, and soy products, and resveratrol, a polyphenol present in red wine and berries, have been shown to stimulate autophagy, offering a dietary means of enhancing this vital process. These nutrients, acting through various signaling pathways, underscore the complexity and adaptability of autophagy as a fundamental component of cellular health.

The interconnection between autophagy and disease processes further illuminates the critical role of this mechanism in maintaining physiological equilibrium. Impaired autophagy has been implicated in a spectrum of age-related conditions, from neurodegenerative disorders such as Alzheimer's and Parkinson's to cardiovascular diseases and cancer. In these contexts, the accumulation of damaged cellular components due to inadequate autophagic activity contributes to cellular dysfunction and the progression of disease.

Conversely, the enhancement of autophagy offers a protective effect, mitigating the impact of aging on cellular integrity and function.

Given the pivotal role of autophagy in health and disease, practical strategies to bolster this cellular renewal process are of paramount interest. Intermittent fasting, by extending the duration between meals, provides a temporal window in which autophagic activity can be maximized. This approach, which mimics the evolutionary conditions under which autophagy evolved as a critical survival mechanism, can be adapted to modern lifestyles through fasting intervals that align with circadian rhythms, optimizing physiological benefits.

In addition to dietary modulation, regular physical activity stands as a cornerstone of autophagy enhancement. Exercise, especially when varied in intensity and duration, stimulates autophagic flux, a measure of the dynamic process of autophagosome formation and degradation. This stimulation is not merely a transient response but can induce lasting adaptations within muscle tissue and beyond, contributing to improved metabolic health and resilience against stress.

Nutritional strategies to support autophagy extend beyond fasting and include the consumption of foods rich in autophagy-modulating nutrients. A diet emphasizing plant-based foods, particularly those high in polyphenols and other bioactive compounds, can support the body's natural detoxification processes by activating autophagy. Such dietary practices, when integrated into a holistic lifestyle approach, underscore the symbiotic relationship between nutrition, physical activity, and cellular health.

In the quest to maintain cellular vitality and stave off the detriments of aging, autophagy emerges as a critical ally. Through informed lifestyle choices that promote this intrinsic cleansing mechanism, individuals can exert a profound influence on their healthspan, optimizing cellular function and enhancing resilience against the diseases of aging. This dynamic interplay between lifestyle and cellular health epitomizes the broader theme of human agency in the pursuit of longevity, where the decisions made today shape the trajectory of health and vitality in the years to come.

THE MIND'S INFLUENCE ON LONGEVITY

The tapestry of human aging is richly interwoven with threads of mental fortitude and adaptability, revealing that the realm of the mind is as pivotal to longevity as the physical body. This chapter unfolds the profound impact of psychological perspectives and emotional resilience on aging, illuminating how a shift in mindset can transform the experience of growing older from a feared inevitability to a journey marked by growth and vitality.

2.1 CULTIVATING A GROWTH MINDSET FOR AGELESS LIVING

The Concept of a Growth Mindset

Carol Dweck's theory of the growth mindset, a concept originating from her extensive research in psychology, posits that individuals who perceive their talents and abilities as malleable are more likely to embrace challenges, persist in the face of setbacks, and achieve higher levels of success compared to those with a fixed mindset, who view their qualities as static and unchangeable. Applied to the domain of aging, this mindset becomes a lens through which the aging process is not seen as a decline but as an opportunity for continual learning and self-improvement.

Overcoming Age-Related Stereotypes

Society often paints aging with a broad brush of decline and diminishment, a perspective that not only permeates our collective consciousness but can seep into our self-perception as we grow older. This internalization manifests as self-imposed limits, where individuals prematurely resign themselves to a life of reduced activity and engagement based on age alone. Challenging these stereotypes requires a conscious effort to redefine what it means to age, focusing on the potential for growth and the accumulation of wisdom rather than loss.

Consider the practice of setting new fitness goals or learning a new language later in life. These endeavors, often associated with youth, stand as testaments to the capacity for growth and adaptation at any age. They serve as practical examples of how breaking free from societal and self-imposed limits can open new avenues for personal development well into our later years.

Strategies for Developing Resilience

Resilience, the ability to recover from difficulties, is a muscle that strengthens with use. Techniques to foster this quality include mindfulness practices, which anchor us in the present moment and cultivate an awareness that can enhance our response to stress and adversity. Regular physical activity, too, bolsters psychological resilience by releasing endorphins that improve mood and reduce feelings of anxiety and depression. Moreover, the act of setting and achieving goals, no matter the scale, reinforces a sense of agency and self-efficacy that is crucial for resilience.

For instance, incorporating a daily walk into one's routine, a simple yet effective form of physical activity reaps physical benefits and provides a structure within which resilience can flourish. By instilling a habit of overcoming inertia to achieve a set goal, this practice mirrors the broader process of resilience-building, where small victories lay the groundwork for greater psychological fortitude.

Success Stories of Late Bloomers

History and contemporary life alike are dotted with examples of individuals who, later in life, reached remarkable heights of achievement and creativity. These late bloomers, as they are often called, defy the conventional timeline of success and underscore the boundless potential for growth and accomplishment at any age. Their stories, from Colonel Sanders founding KFC in his sixties to Grandma Moses beginning her painting career in her late seventies, serve as an inspiration and concrete evidence of the growth mindset in action.

These narratives share a common thread: a refusal to allow age to define capability. They remind us that the barriers we perceive around aging are often of our own making and that the capacity for achievement and fulfillment extends far beyond societal expectations.

Reflective Exercise: Envisioning Growth at Every Age

Consider a goal or aspiration you have yet to pursue, possibly deterred by the belief that it's "too late." Write it down, detailing why it holds importance for you and the steps you could take to achieve it, however small. This exercise is about more than immediate success but about reorienting your perspective towards growth and possibility, regardless of age.

In the realm of aging, where society often emphasizes limitation, cultivating a growth mindset offers a powerful counter-narrative. It challenges us to view each year not as a step toward decline but as an opportunity for continued development, learning, and resilience. When nurtured and applied, this mindset becomes a key determinant of how we experience aging, transforming it into a period rich with potential for personal evolution and fulfillment.

2.2 THE LINK BETWEEN EMOTIONAL HEALTH AND LONGEVITY

Emotional well-being occupies a central role in the intricate dance of longevity, where the harmonies and discord of our inner emotional landscapes play a pivotal part in shaping the contours of our life span. Groundbreaking research has laid bare a compelling connection between the states of our emotional health and the lengths of our lives, unveiling a truth that underscores the profound impact of emotional well-being on our physical existence. Studies, such as those cataloged in the *American Journal of Epidemiology*, reveal that individuals exhibiting positive emotional attributes like contentment, happiness, and enthusiasm are less susceptible to premature mortality than their less content counterparts. This correlation highlights the significance of emotional health as a critical component of longevity. It sets the stage for a deeper inquiry into the mechanisms through which emotional states influence our biological processes.

Navigating the terrain of emotional wellness necessitates a toolkit brimming with practical methods designed to mitigate stress, anxiety, and depression—common afflictions that, if left unchecked, can erode the foundations of our emotional and physical health. Mindfulness meditation emerges as a potent tool in this arsenal, offering a pathway to tranquility through the cultivation of present-moment awareness. This ancient practice, rooted in Buddhist traditions and validated by contemporary science, encourages a non-judgmental observation of thoughts and feelings, thereby fostering a state of calm detachment that can significantly lower stress levels. Cognitive-behavioral therapy (CBT), another cornerstone in the edifice of emotional wellness, empowers individuals with strategies to reframe negative thought patterns, thereby alleviating the symptoms of anxiety and depression. By equipping individuals with the means to challenge and change maladaptive thinking, CBT lays the groundwork for a more resilient and emotionally balanced life.

The role of social connections in fortifying our emotional defenses against the vicissitudes of aging cannot be overstated. A wealth of evidence underscores the link between robust social networks and enhanced longevity, painting a vivid picture of human interconnectedness as a vital lifeline. Research delineated in the journal *Psychosomatic Medicine* elucidates how strong, supportive relationships act as buffers against the stressors that can compromise our health, reducing the risk of chronic conditions such as heart disease and bolstering immune system function. These findings illuminate the profound impact of social bonds on our well-being, suggesting that the quality and depth of our relationships are integral to our longevity.

Fostering a supportive emotional environment becomes an endeavor of paramount importance. Cultivating such an environment requires a deliberate effort to nurture relationships that provide emotional sustenance through family ties, friendships, or community connections. This process involves reaching out, deepening existing relationships, and expanding one's social horizon by engaging in group activities, volunteering, or joining clubs that align with personal interests. These interactions, rich with the potential for emotional exchange and growth, create a scaffolding of support that can sustain us through the challenges and transitions inherent in aging.

Moreover, the act of giving and receiving emotional support within these networks engenders a sense of belonging and purpose, elements that are inextricably linked to emotional well-being. Initiatives such as peer support groups for older adults or mentorship programs that leverage the wisdom of age in guiding the younger generation can amplify these benefits, creating a reciprocal flow of support that enriches all involved. Through these channels, individuals find solace and understanding and opportunities to contribute meaningfully to the lives of others, thereby reinforcing their sense of value and self-worth.

In exploring the nexus between emotional health and longevity, it becomes evident that the journey toward a longer, healthier life is as much about nurturing the heart and soul as it is about caring for the body. The tapestry of longevity, with its myriad threads of physical and emotional well-being, weaves a narrative that speaks to the holistic nature of health. In attending to our emotional landscapes with the same diligence we afford our physical bodies, we open ourselves to a broader spectrum of wellness that embraces the fullness of our human experience. Through the cultivation of emotional resilience, the deepening of social connections, and the creation of supportive environments, we lay the groundwork for a life marked not only by length but by richness and fulfillment. This approach, grounded in recognizing emotional health as a cornerstone of longevity, charts a course for a future in which aging is not a process of decline but a continuing journey of growth and discovery.

2.3 OVERCOMING AGE-RELATED MENTAL HEALTH CHALLENGES

Within the panorama of aging, the emergence of mental health issues such as depression, anxiety, and loneliness cast shadows that can obscure the vibrancy of later life. These challenges, prevalent among aging populations, demand attention for their frequency and profound impact on quality of life. Identifying these conditions becomes crucial, a step that necessitates vigilance and awareness from individuals and those within their circles. Depression, with its cloak of pervasive sadness and disinterest, often masquerades as a natural component of aging, yet it is anything but. Anxiety, too, presents a formidable obstacle, manifesting through undue worries and fears that can constrict daily living. Loneliness, an epidemic in its own right, exacerbates these conditions, creating a cycle that can spiral without intervention.

The pathway to mitigating these mental health challenges is multifaceted, beginning with the crucial step of accessing resources and support. The landscape of assistance is diverse, encompassing professional help from psychologists and psychiatrists whose expertise can guide individuals through the maze of mental health struggles. Yet, beyond the realm of professional intervention lies a network of community resources and support groups, spaces where individuals can find solace and understanding among peers navigating similar challenges. These groups, often facilitated by organizations dedicated to senior well-being, offer not just companionship but practical strategies for coping grounded in shared experiences and communal wisdom.

In tandem with these resources, mindfulness and cognitive behavioral strategies emerge as potent tools for reclaiming mental equilibrium. Mindfulness, the practice of anchoring oneself in the present moment with acceptance and without judgment, offers a refuge from the tumult of anxious thoughts and depressive ruminations. Through techniques such as focused breathing and mindful meditation, individuals learn to observe their mental landscape with detachment, reducing the intensity of negative emotions and fostering a sense of peace. Cognitive-behavioral therapy (CBT), focusing on altering dysfunctional thought patterns, provides a complementary approach. This strategy empowers individuals to challenge and reframe cognitive distortions—such as the tendency to magnify negatives or to overgeneralize from singular events— thereby diluting the potency of anxiety and depression.

Promoting mental health through lifestyle adjustments offers another avenue for addressing age-related mental challenges. Nutrition plays a subtle yet significant role in this regard. Diets rich in omega-3 fatty acids, antioxidants, and vitamins, found in foods such as fatty fish, berries, nuts, and leafy greens, support brain health and can mitigate symptoms of depression and anxiety. Physical exercise, too, stands as a cornerstone of mental well-being. Activities such as walking, yoga, and tai chi enhance physical health and release endorphins that act as natural mood elevators, fostering a sense of well-being. Beyond diet and exercise, engagement in hobbies and pursuits that nourish the soul—be it through art, music, gardening, or volunteer work—injects a sense of purpose and joy into daily life, counteracting feelings of loneliness and the existential ennui that can accompany aging.

This approach to confronting mental health challenges in aging is not a quick fix but a sustained effort, one that acknowledges the complexity of the human psyche and the varied tools required to navigate its waters. By recognizing the prevalence of these issues, seeking out appropriate resources and support, employing mindfulness and cognitive strategies, and making targeted lifestyle adjustments, individuals can illuminate the shadows cast by mental health challenges, revealing a landscape of aging marked not by decline but by resilience and a deepened capacity for joy.

2.4 HARNESSING THE POWER OF RESILIENCE AND ADAPTABILITY

In the vast landscape of human experience, resilience stands as a beacon, illuminating the path through the trials and tribulations of life. This quality, particularly poignant in the context of aging, embodies the capacity to recover and flourish in the face of adversity. It is not merely about enduring but thriving amidst the challenges that life unfurls. The essence of resilience lies in the alchemy of transforming hardship into growth, a process that is both universal and deeply personal.

The cultivation of resilience is akin to tending a garden. It requires patience, care, and the right conditions to flourish. Mindfulness practice is one such tool, a method by which individuals can cultivate a centered presence, observing their experiences with compassion and detachment. This practice roots the mind in the present, providing a stable foundation to face life's storms. Gratitude, another vital practice, acts as sunlight, nourishing the soul with a focus on abundance rather than lack. This shift in perspective fosters resilience by highlighting the gifts within each moment, even in hardship. Physical activity, too, strengthens the body and mind, reinforcing the physical vessel through which resilience manifests. Though simple in concept, each of these practices requires consistent application to yield the fruits of resilience.

Adaptability, a close kin to resilience, speaks to the capacity to navigate the winds of change with grace and flexibility. It is the skill of adjusting one's sails to the shifting winds of life, finding new directions and possibilities in the face of change. This quality is vital as one ages, a period often marked by significant transitions and adjustments. The essence of adaptability lies in the recognition that change is not only inevitable but also a fertile ground for growth and renewal. It is an invitation to view each new phase of life not as a loss but as an opportunity to explore, learn, and redefine oneself.

The lives of those who embody resilience and adaptability offer a wellspring of inspiration. Consider the story of a woman who, after decades in a fulfilling career, faced retirement not as the end but as a new chapter. She turned to painting, a passion she had long deferred, finding in it a new source of joy and meaning. Her story reflects the resilience to redefine her identity in the face of change and the adaptability to embrace new pursuits enthusiastically. Another case is that of a man who, after the loss of his spouse, transformed his grief into action by founding a community group for fellow widowers. His journey illustrates resilience in the face of profound loss and adaptability in creating a new sense of purpose through service.

These stories, and countless others like them, underscore the transformative power of resilience and adaptability. They demonstrate that aging, far from being a decline, can be a time of profound growth and reinvention. Cultivating these qualities is not a passive process but an active engagement with life, a conscious choice to grow and thrive regardless of circumstances.

As we turn the page on this exploration of resilience and adaptability, we are reminded of the indomitable spirit that resides within each of us. The journey through life, with its inevitable ups and downs, offers endless opportunities to strengthen these qualities. By embracing mindfulness, gratitude, and physical activity as tools for resilience and by viewing change as a gateway to new possibilities, we can navigate the challenges of aging with courage and grace.

This chapter in our lives, far from signaling a diminishment, can be a time of unparalleled growth, a testament to the enduring capacity of the human spirit to evolve and flourish.

In the chapters that follow, we will continue to explore the myriad dimensions of wellness and longevity, each thread weaving into the next, creating a tapestry rich with insight and guidance for a life lived to its fullest.

NOURISHING LONGEVITY: THE POWER OF DIET

In the mosaic of factors contributing to a long and healthy life, diet holds a pivotal role, a thread weaving through the fabric of wellness with patterns as diverse as they are profound. The adage "You are what you eat" resonates with heightened significance as we examine the intricate dance between nutrition and aging. This chapter delves into the heart of dietary practices that promise not just years to life but life to years, exploring the alchemy of foods that defy the aging process and the myths that cloud our nutritional choices.

3.1 THE LONGEVITY DIET: FOODS THAT FIGHT AGING

Principles of the Longevity Diet

The longevity diet emerges from a synthesis of research spanning cultures, continents, and centuries, revealing a common thread: a pattern of eating that emphasizes whole, nutrient-dense foods. This diet is not a prescriptive regimen but a flexible framework, accommodating a tapestry of dietary habits grounded in the consumption of vegetables, fruits, whole grains, legumes, nuts, and seeds, with minimal reliance on processed foods. The Mediterranean diet, rich in olive oil, fish, and an abundance of fresh produce, exemplifies these principles and stands as a beacon of dietary wisdom, with its followers enjoying markedly lower rates of chronic diseases and extended lifespans.

Imagine walking through a bustling local farmer's market on a crisp Saturday morning, your senses awakened by the vibrant colors and earthy scents of fresh produce. This simple act of choosing locally grown, seasonal foods can be a cornerstone of the longevity diet, a practice that supports sustainable agriculture and ensures a diet rich in the antioxidants, fibers, and phytonutrients essential for cellular health and longevity.

Anti-aging Nutrients and Foods

The quest for the fountain of youth may lead not to a mythical spring but to the grocery aisle, where a plethora of foods laden with anti-aging properties awaits. Omega-3 fatty acids, found in abundance in fatty fish like salmon and in flaxseeds, wield anti-inflammatory powers that combat the chronic inflammation underlying many age-related diseases. Berries, with their rich anthocyanin content, offer antioxidant protection against cellular damage, while nuts, a treasure trove of healthy fats, vitamins, and minerals, support brain health and cardiovascular function.

The narrative of anti-aging nutrients is incomplete without a nod to the humble spice turmeric, its active compound curcumin lauded for its potent anti-inflammatory and antioxidant effects. Incorporating turmeric into daily meals, perhaps through a warming golden milk latte or a vibrant curry, can be a simple yet effective strategy for harnessing its health benefits.

Incorporating Longevity Foods into Daily Meals

Incorporating longevity-promoting foods into everyday meals is an art that demands both creativity and a conscious effort. Let's envision a day's menu crafted to seamlessly weave these nutrient-rich foods into each meal. For breakfast, imagine a vibrant smoothie bowl as the canvas, richly painted with a blend of mixed berries known for their antioxidant prowess, sprinkled with chia seeds for that fiber and omega-3 boost, and finished with a generous swirl of almond butter for healthy fats and a touch of luxury. Transitioning to lunch, a quinoa salad becomes the stage for a symphony of textures and tastes. This salad is abundant with leafy greens, providing a wealth of vitamins and minerals, mixed with chickpeas for a hearty dose of protein and fiber, all brought together with a lavish drizzle of olive oil, celebrating the heart-healthy monounsaturated fats. As the day wanes, dinner embraces the Mediterranean ethos, a tradition celebrated for its longevity-promoting diet. Picture a beautifully grilled salmon, its omega-3 fatty acids a beacon of anti-inflammatory benefits, accompanied by a side of roasted vegetables, their edges caramelized and flavors intensified, offering a bounty of antioxidants. A simple salad on the side, dressed lightly, provides a crisp and refreshing counterpoint, making each meal a moment of nourishment and a mosaic of flavors and nutrients designed to protect and invigorate the body. Through this detailed daily meal plan, we see that integrating foods that promote longevity into our diet can be both delicious and deeply fulfilling, a testament to the idea that what is good for us can also be a source of joy and satisfaction.

Debunking Diet Myths

In the realm of nutrition, myths and misconceptions abound, casting shadows of doubt over time-honored dietary wisdom. The vilification of fats as a universal foe overlooks the nuanced reality of dietary lipids, where the type and quality of fat—such as the monounsaturated fats in avocados and olive oil—matter more than quantity. Similarly, the demonization of carbohydrates fails to distinguish between the refined sugars and flours driving metabolic dysfunction and the complex carbohydrates in whole grains and legumes that fuel our bodies with sustained energy and fiber. Proteins, too, are often entangled in debates that obscure the value of plant-based sources like lentils and tempeh, which offer a bounty of nutrients beyond amino acids.

In navigating these myths, the wisdom of moderation and diversity becomes clear. A diet that embraces a variety of whole foods, balancing macronutrients and flavors, emerges as a blueprint for longevity. This approach, grounded in the principles of the longevity diet, transcends the cacophony of dietary trends, guiding us toward a way of eating that is as enriching as nourishing.

Visual Element: The Longevity Diet Plate

A vibrant infographic, "The Longevity Diet Plate," offers a visual guide to constructing meals that embody the principles of the longevity diet. This plate is divided into colorful segments, each representing a vital component of the diet—fruits, vegetables, whole grains, healthy proteins, and fats—with portion sizes and examples provided. Accompanying the infographic, a checklist of anti-aging superfoods encourages readers to explore the diversity of nutrient-rich foods, making each meal an adventure in healthful eating.

By embracing the longevity diet, we engage in a daily practice of self-care that honors our bodies' needs and the profound connection between diet and wellness. This chapter invites readers to look beyond the fleeting allure of dietary fads, finding solace and vitality in the timeless wisdom of whole, life-affirming foods.

3.2 SUPERFOODS FOR SUPERIOR HEALTH: BEYOND THE HYPE

In the realm of nutrition, the term "superfoods" often sparkles with a sheen of promise, suggesting a category of edibles endowed with an almost magical efficacy in enhancing health and vitality. These are foods distinguished not by esoteric qualities or inaccessible rarity but by their dense concentration of vitamins, minerals, antioxidants, and other nutrients critical for robust health. The true power of superfoods lies in their ability to deliver these essential nutrients in natural, whole-food forms, making them a vital cornerstone of any diet aimed at promoting longevity and warding off disease.

Exploring the landscape of superfoods unveils a spectrum that extends far beyond the familiar staples of avocados, blueberries, and kale, reaching into a treasury of underappreciated gems that pack a nutritional punch. Consider the humble moringa leaf, often dubbed "the miracle tree," which thrives in arid climates. Its leaves are a powerhouse of nutrition, rich in calcium, iron, and essential amino acids, offering a potent supplement to diets where such nutrients are scarce. Similarly, the baobab fruit, native to Africa, bursts with antioxidants, vitamin C, and prebiotic fiber; its tangy pulp is a versatile ingredient for boosting the nutritional profile of smoothies and sauces.

The wisdom of traditional diets, honed over generations, has long recognized the value of what the modern lexicon terms as superfoods. Maca root has been utilized for centuries in the high Andean plateaus for its remarkable stamina and energy-boosting properties. Across the Pacific, in the traditional Japanese diet, seaweeds like nori and wakame are celebrated not only for their umami flavor but for their rich content of iodine and tyrosine, which are crucial for thyroid health. These practices are not remnants of a bygone era but living testimonies to the enduring relevance of superfoods in sustaining health and longevity.

Incorporating these nutritional titans into contemporary diets necessitates creativity and an openness to new flavors and textures. Infusing daily meals with these superfoods can be as simple as sprinkling chia seeds, rich in omega-3 fatty acids and fiber, over morning oatmeal or blending spirulina, a potent source of plant-based protein and essential vitamins, into a post-workout smoothie. The art of modern cooking has evolved to embrace these ingredients, transforming them from mere nutritional supplements to stars of the culinary show. A salad becomes a canvas for a rainbow of superfoods; quinoa, pomegranate seeds, and roasted nuts dressed with a turmeric vinaigrette create a symphony of flavors that nourish the body and delight the palate.

To be candid, navigating the dietary aspect of my wellness and longevity journey has presented its challenges. My palate doesn't naturally align with many foods traditionally highlighted in the Mediterranean diet, a fact that underscores the importance of creativity in this lifelong endeavor. Rather than focusing on the foods that don't appeal to me, such as most fish and leafy greens, I've turned my attention to the vibrant world of fruits, seeds, and nuts. It's a testament to the idea that wellness journeys are highly personal and subject to adaptation. Flexibility, assessment, and finding joy in the alternatives are crucial. With patience and an open mind, it's possible to tailor dietary choices that not only meet nutritional needs but also fit personal tastes. Embarking on this exploration of superfoods, from the ancient grains of the Andes to the nourishing sea vegetables of the Pacific, highlights a fundamental principle: the most effective tools for health and longevity are often not found in modern pharmacies but in our own kitchens and pantries. The process of selecting, preparing, and enjoying these nutrient-rich foods is an intimate connection to centuries of tradition and wisdom. This journey reveals that achieving superior health goes beyond the trends and fads, grounding itself in a deep appreciation for the sustenance provided by our planet.

3.3 NAVIGATING DIETARY SUPPLEMENTS FOR AGING ADULTS

In the intricate tapestry of nutritional wellness that adorns the landscape of aging, dietary supplements emerge as both allies and enigmas. Their role, woven between the threads of whole foods and balanced diets, offers a nuanced layer of support to the aging body, addressing gaps and bolstering health where diet alone may fall short. This segment delves into the nuanced considerations surrounding supplements, guiding through the labyrinth of choices to illuminate paths backed by scientific rigor and marked by safety.

Amidst the evolving narrative of aging, the question of when and why supplements become necessary punctuates the discourse with urgency and caution. With advancing years, the body's ability to absorb nutrients from food diminishes, a reality further compounded by increased nutritional needs and the prevalence of chronic conditions. In this context, supplements serve not as replacements but as strategic reinforcements, filling nutritional voids that could otherwise widen into health chasms. This supplementation is particularly critical for vitamins D and B12, calcium, and omega-3 fatty acids, nutrients essential for maintaining bone density, cognitive function, and cardiovascular health, yet often deficient in older adults.

Selecting the right supplements, however, demands discernment. The criteria for this selection process prioritize purity, potency, and bioavailability. High-quality supplements, devoid of unnecessary fillers and additives, ensure that the body receives the intended nutrients without the burden of processing extraneous substances. Potency, indicating the concentration of active ingredients, must align with established guidelines for daily intake, avoiding the pitfalls of under- or over-supplementation. Bioavailability, the extent to which a nutrient is absorbed and utilized by the body, becomes a critical factor, steering towards forms of supplements that offer maximum benefit. Third-party certifications from organizations like the US Pharmacopeia (USP) or ConsumerLab provide an additional layer of assurance, attesting to the supplement's quality and efficacy.

Yet, the landscape of supplementation is not without its hazards. Potential risks and interactions with medications loom as significant concerns, underscoring the importance of informed choices. Over-supplementation, particularly with fat-soluble vitamins such as A, D, E, and K, invites the risk of toxicity, as these nutrients accumulate in the body's tissues over time. Furthermore, the interplay between supplements and prescription medications can alter drug efficacy or precipitate adverse reactions, a risk particularly acute with blood thinners and supplements like ginkgo biloba or high doses of omega-3 fatty acids. This delicate balance necessitates a dialogue between individuals and healthcare professionals, ensuring that supplement regimens complement rather than complicate medical treatments.

In the pursuit of supplements backed by science, certain nutrients stand out for their evidence-based benefits to aging populations. Vitamin D, often dubbed the "sunshine vitamin," commands attention for its role in bone health and immune function, with supplementation proving beneficial in mitigating deficiency and supporting overall health in older adults. Omega-3 fatty acids, derived from fish oil supplements, are lauded for their cardiovascular benefits and potential to reduce inflammation, a cornerstone of many age-related diseases. Probiotics are live microorganisms that confer health benefits when administered in adequate amounts, support gut health and are a critical component of immune function and nutrient absorption. Magnesium, involved in over 300 biochemical reactions in the body, merits consideration for its contributions to muscle function, sleep quality, and metabolic health, areas of concern for many as they age.

Beyond these, coenzyme Q10 (CoQ10), an antioxidant supporting cellular energy production and heart health, and curcumin, the active component in turmeric known for its anti-inflammatory properties, embody the convergence of traditional wisdom and modern science. These supplements, among others, offer tangible benefits rooted in rigorous research, providing strategic support in the multifaceted endeavor of aging well.

Vitamin D, Ginger, and Lion's Mane have all been beneficial among the supplements I've explored. However, turmeric stood out for its profound impact on my health, particularly in fighting inflammation. Initially, my experience with turmeric was marred by its harsh effects on my stomach, leading me to discontinue its use. This setback prompted further investigation into anti-inflammatory supplements, where turmeric's benefits were consistently highlighted. Recognizing the necessity to incorporate turmeric into my regimen, I sought solutions to its digestive challenges. Conversations with others revealed a common strategy for mitigating these adverse effects: combining turmeric with milk or yogurt. By adopting this method, I was able to reintroduce turmeric into my daily supplement regimen, making it an essential component of my health protocol.

Navigating the nuanced terrain of dietary supplements for aging adults involves the interplay of necessity, quality, safety, and scientific backing. This journey, marked by personal health histories and future aspirations, emphasizes supplements as components of a broader strategy encompassing diet, lifestyle, and preventive healthcare. As individuals traverse this landscape, the choices made today in the realm of supplementation hold the promise of enhancing vitality and well-being in the years to come, each selection a step towards a future of sustained health and longevity.

3.4 INTERMITTENT FASTING AND CIRCADIAN RHYTHMS

Within the domain of nutritional science, intermittent fasting emerges as a paradigm that redefines our engagement with food, not through the prism of what we eat but when we eat. This practice, which alternates intervals of eating with periods of fasting, taps into the primal machinery of our metabolism, evoking a spectrum of physiological responses that echo the ancient rhythms of feast and famine. The essence of intermittent fasting lies in its flexibility, encompassing various protocols such as the 16/8 method, where sixteen hours of fasting give way to an eight-hour eating window, and the 5:2 approach, which advocates for normal eating for five days juxtaposed against a caloric restriction on two non-consecutive days. Each method activates a cascade of metabolic processes, from the mobilization of fat stores for energy to the enhancement of cellular repair mechanisms, illustrating the profound adaptability of the human body to temporal patterns of nutrient intake.

The symbiosis between intermittent fasting and circadian rhythms, the internal clock that orchestrates our physiological functions, presents a compelling narrative in the pursuit of optimal health. Circadian rhythms, attuned to the daily cycle of light and darkness, govern an array of biological processes, including hormone release, sleep-wake cycles, and metabolism. Aligning eating patterns with these rhythms by confining food intake to daylight hours, for instance, optimizes metabolic efficiency, ensuring that food is consumed and processed when the body is primed for digestion and nutrient absorption. This alignment, which mirrors the eating patterns of our ancestors, who were bound by the natural light cycles, minimizes metabolic disruptions, fostering an environment conducive to weight management, improved sleep quality, and overall metabolic health.

The merits of intermittent fasting extend into aging, where its impact manifests in the attenuation of age-related decline. The mechanism through which fasting exerts its beneficial effects is multifaceted. It involves reducing oxidative stress, improving insulin sensitivity, and initiating autophagy, the cellular clean-up process that removes damaged components. These processes collectively contribute to an enhanced metabolic profile, reduced inflammation, and improved brain function, laying a foundation for a resilient aging process. Furthermore, intermittent fasting has been shown to stimulate the production of neurotrophic factors, which support neuronal growth and cognitive function, offering a buffer against neurodegenerative disorders.

Adapting intermittent fasting to one's lifestyle demands a personalized approach that considers individual health status, lifestyle factors, and personal preferences. Initiating this practice with gradual adjustments, such as extending the overnight fasting period by delaying breakfast or advancing dinner time, can ease the transition, minimizing discomfort and enhancing adherence. Monitoring one's response to fasting, both physically and mentally, allows for fine-tuning of fasting intervals to align with personal health goals and lifestyle demands. Notably, during eating windows, focusing on nutrient-dense foods that provide essential vitamins, minerals, and antioxidants ensures that the body receives the nourishment it needs to thrive under this regimen.

For those embarking on this path, consulting with healthcare professionals ensures that intermittent fasting is undertaken safely, particularly for individuals with existing health conditions or those on medication. This dialogue is crucial in tailoring the fasting approach to individual health needs, mitigating potential risks, and maximizing the benefits of this dietary strategy.

In closing, intermittent fasting stands not merely as a dietary trend but as a testament to the human body's adaptability and its innate capacity for health and longevity. By weaving the principles of intermittent fasting with the natural cadence of our circadian rhythms, we tap into a powerful synergy that supports metabolic health, cognitive function, and cellular repair. While exploring the contours of intermittent fasting, this chapter uncovers a broader narrative of nutritional science that embraces the human body's complexity and its remarkable capacity for resilience and renewal. As we transition from the exploration of dietary strategies, the journey continues towards a deeper understanding of movement and physical activity, integral components of a holistic approach to longevity.

MOVEMENT AS MEDICINE

The human body thrives on movement; it is its language, a form of expression connected to the essence of life itself. In the same way that a river carves its path through the landscape, so too does physical activity shape the contours of our health. This chapter uncovers the profound relationship between exercise and the aging process, offering insights into how tailored physical activity becomes a pivotal ally in the pursuit of longevity.

4.1 TAILORING YOUR EXERCISE REGIMEN TO YOUR AGE

Assessing Fitness Levels

Before embarking on any fitness program, understanding one's starting point is crucial. This involves evaluating physical capabilities and recognizing limitations, a process akin to mapping the terrain before a hike. The first step is a self-assessment, which could be as simple as noting how many flights of stairs can be climbed without pause or how long one can walk before feeling fatigued.

For a more structured approach, consulting with a fitness professional who can conduct assessments such as flexibility tests, cardiovascular fitness evaluations, and strength measurements offers invaluable insights. This baseline not only informs the design of the exercise program but also serves as a reference point for measuring progress.

Creating a Balanced Exercise Program

A well-rounded exercise regimen is the cornerstone of fitness at any age, embodying a harmony between cardiovascular, strength, flexibility, and balance training. Each component plays a unique role: cardiovascular exercises, like walking or cycling, improve heart health and endurance; strength training, using resistance bands or weights, builds muscle and bone density; flexibility exercises increase the range of motion, reducing the risk of injury; and balance exercises prevent falls, a common concern as we age. A balanced program might look like alternating cardio days with strength training, incorporating flexibility exercises at the end of each session, and dedicating specific days to balance-focused activities. This multifaceted approach ensures comprehensive benefits, addressing the diverse needs of the aging body.

Adapting Exercises for Safety and Effectiveness

Modifying exercises ensures they are safe and effective for older adults. For instance, chair squats can be a safer alternative to traditional squats, providing stability while still targeting the major muscle groups of the legs. Similarly, low-impact exercises such as swimming or water aerobics reduce joint stress while offering cardiovascular and strength benefits. These adaptations are not about diminishing the exercise's value but about customizing the approach to align with the individual's physical condition, maximizing benefits while minimizing risks.

Setting and Achieving Fitness Goals

Setting realistic, achievable goals is vital for maintaining motivation and tracking progress. Goals should be specific, measurable, attainable, relevant, and time-bound (SMART). For example, aiming to walk 30 minutes a day, five days a week, is a clear and measurable goal. Recording these activities in a journal or app not only aids in tracking progress but also in recognizing achievements, no matter how small. Celebrating these milestones fosters a sense of accomplishment, fueling motivation to continue pursuing higher levels of fitness.

Visual Element: Exercise Modification Chart

An infographic titled "Exercise Modifications for Aging Adults" visually presents alternatives to common exercises, making the information accessible and practical. This chart details modifications for exercises such as squats, lunges, and push-ups, offering variations that decrease joint strain while ensuring the exercise remains beneficial. Accompanying each modification, icons indicate the primary muscle groups targeted, providing a quick reference for incorporating these adaptations into workout routines.

In understanding the symbiotic relationship between movement and aging, it becomes evident that exercise is not merely a tool for maintaining physical health but a vital component of living fully at any age. By assessing individual fitness levels, crafting a balanced and varied exercise program, adapting activities for safety, and setting attainable goals, the groundwork is laid for a lifestyle that embraces activity as both a joy and a necessity. This chapter, dedicated to unraveling the complexities of tailoring exercise to the aging body, illuminates the path toward a future where movement and medicine merge, unlocking the potential for a life marked not by the years but by the vitality within them.

4.2 THE SCIENCE OF STRENGTH TRAINING FOR SENIORS

Strength training, often perceived as the domain of the young and robust, holds profound implications for the senior population, challenging the misconception that it leads to undue strain and injury in an aging body. This form of physical conditioning emphasizes the use of resistance to induce muscular contraction and builds strength, anaerobic endurance, and the size of skeletal muscles. For seniors, these outcomes translate into not only an enhanced quality of life but also a formidable defense against the ravages of aging.

The skeletal system, a living structure that remodels itself throughout life, responds to the stresses placed upon it in a manner akin to muscle adaptation under resistance training. This process, known as bone modeling, thrives under the weight-bearing exercises of strength training, which stimulate bone-forming cells and slow the loss of bone density. Consequently, the risk of osteoporosis, a condition marked by weakened bones and heightened fracture risk, diminishes significantly. Furthermore, the accrual of muscle mass through regular strength-oriented workouts counteracts sarcopenia, the natural decline of muscle tissue with age, thereby preserving mobility and independence. Metabolic health, too, sees remarkable improvements as strength training elevates resting metabolic rate, aiding in the management of body weight and composition and enhancing glucose regulation, a critical factor in preventing and managing type 2 diabetes.

Implementing safe strength training practices for seniors hinges on adherence to proper form and the careful selection of resistance levels. Mastery of form, precise alignment, and movement during exercise safeguard against the undue strain that can lead to injuries. This mastery begins with a focus on low weights or even body-weight exercises, gradually increasing resistance only as strength and confidence build. The guidance of certified trainers, especially in the initial stages, can provide personalized instruction, ensuring exercises are performed with the correct form. Furthermore, the choice of weights must reflect the individual's current strength levels, avoiding the common pitfall of overestimation that leads to muscle strain or injury. Emphasis on slow, controlled movements enhances muscle activation and minimizes risk, making strength training a safe and effective component of a senior's fitness regimen.

The debate between the merits of home-based versus gym-based routines for strength training in seniors presents multiple considerations. Home environments, with the aid of minimal equipment such as resistance bands, light dumbbells, and stability balls, offer a convenient and comfortable setting for many seniors, reducing barriers to regular exercise. Additionally, the privacy of home-based routines can alleviate the intimidation or self-consciousness often felt by seniors in gym settings. Conversely, gyms provide access to a broader range of equipment and the opportunity for social interaction, which can motivate and enhance the exercise experience. Therefore, the choice between home and gym environments rests on personal preferences, goals, and the availability of resources, underscoring the flexibility of strength training as a modality adaptable to diverse lifestyles and needs.

Narratives of seniors who have woven strength training into the fabric of their lives resonate with transformation and empowerment. Take, for instance, the story of a 72-year-old who, after years of leading a sedentary lifestyle, discovered strength training and gradually built up her physical capabilities, eventually participating in her first strength competition. Her journey, marked by initial hesitations and gradual triumphs, highlights not only the physical transformations possible through strength training but also the profound impact on self-esteem and mental well-being. Another narrative unfolds from a senior who integrated strength exercises into his routine following a diagnosis of osteopenia, a precursor to osteoporosis. Over time, his dedication not only halted the progression of bone density loss but reversed it, demonstrating the capacity of strength training to directly confront and alter the course of age-related health challenges.

These stories, emblematic of countless others, illuminate the transformative potential of strength training for seniors. This practice transcends physical benefits to touch upon the deeper realms of confidence, resilience, and autonomy. They underscore the message that age, far from being a barrier to physical improvement, offers a unique opportunity for renewal and growth.

Strength training for seniors, with its myriad benefits from improved bone density and muscle mass to better metabolic health, emerges not just as a strategy for maintaining physical function but as a powerful means of enhancing life's quality and duration. Through careful attention to form, appropriate weight selection, and the choice between home or gym settings, seniors can safely and effectively engage in strength training, reaping its rewards. The narratives of those who have embarked on this path of physical conditioning in their later years serve not only as a testament to its feasibility but as beacons of inspiration, proving that strength, both physical and inner, knows no age limit.

4.3 LOW-IMPACT WORKOUTS: EFFECTIVE OPTIONS FOR EVERY FITNESS LEVEL

Navigating the landscape of physical activity reveals a multitude of paths, with low-impact exercises emerging as a gentle yet potent modality tailored to the nuanced needs of individuals across the spectrum of fitness levels. These activities, characterized by minimal stress on the body's joints, offer a sanctuary for those seeking to maintain or enhance their physical health without the risk of injury inherent in more strenuous forms of exercise. Among the myriad options available, walking stands out for its simplicity and accessibility. It demands no specialized equipment nor the confines of a gym, providing the freedom to engage with the natural world directly. The rhythmic cadence of footsteps, whether on a forest trail or urban sidewalk, not only fortifies cardiovascular health but also serves as a meditative practice, clearing the mind and elevating mood.

Swimming, by contrast, offers a buoyant embrace that liberates the body from the constraints of gravity, allowing for a comprehensive workout that feels deceptively effortless. This aquatic exercise engages multiple muscle groups simultaneously, enhancing muscular endurance and flexibility while the water's resistance ensures a cardiovascular challenge. For individuals grappling with arthritis or recovering from injury, the supportive environment of water reduces pain and facilitates movement, making swimming a particularly inclusive form of low-impact exercise.

Cycling, whether pursued outdoors on winding paths and scenic routes or indoors on stationary bikes, presents another avenue for low-impact cardiovascular improvement. The cyclic motion, propelling the bike forward, demands engagement from the legs, core, and cardiovascular system, offering a balanced workout that spares the joints from harsh impacts. Additionally, the variable resistance and speed allow for customization according to individual fitness levels, ensuring a challenging yet manageable exercise experience.

Yoga, a practice steeped in ancient tradition, transcends the boundaries of mere physical activity to encompass a holistic approach to well-being. Through a series of postures and controlled breathing techniques, yoga cultivates not only flexibility and balance but also a deep sense of mental and emotional tranquility. Each pose, from the grounding stability of the mountain pose to the gentle stretch of the downward dog, is an exploration of the body's potential, adaptable to varying degrees of flexibility and strength. Moreover, yoga's emphasis on mindfulness and breath awareness integrates a dimension of mental health benefits, making it a multifaceted tool in the quest for holistic wellness.

Designing a low-impact workout routine requires more than the selection of activities; it demands a thoughtful integration of variety and progression to avoid the plateaus often encountered in fitness journeys. A week might intersperse days of walking with sessions of swimming or cycling, incorporating yoga on alternate days to ensure a balanced engagement of the body's various muscle groups. This variety not only prevents the monotony that can dampen motivation but also ensures a comprehensive approach to fitness, addressing cardiovascular health, muscular strength, flexibility, and balance in equal measure.

Progression, the gradual increase in the duration, frequency, or intensity of workouts, ensures that the body continues to adapt and evolve in response to physical activity. For instance, incrementally extending the distance of walks or the length of swimming sessions challenges the body, enhancing endurance. Similarly, exploring more advanced yoga poses or adding resistance to cycling routines can elevate the workout's intensity, fostering continued improvement in fitness levels.

Overcoming barriers to regular exercise, particularly those encountered by individuals engaging in low-impact workouts hinges on strategies that address both the physical and psychological facets of fitness. For some, the perceived lack of challenge in low-impact exercises can diminish motivation. In these instances, setting clear, measurable goals related to distance, duration, or flexibility can imbue these activities with a sense of purpose and achievement. For others, physical limitations or discomfort may pose significant obstacles. Here, adapting exercises to accommodate individual needs, such as using props in yoga or adjusting the seat height on a bicycle, can mitigate discomfort and enhance the enjoyment of the activity.

Social support plays a critical role in sustaining motivation. Joining walking groups, enrolling in group swim sessions, or participating in community yoga classes can provide camaraderie and account-ability, making the commitment to regular exercise a shared endeavor. For those who prefer the solitude of solo workouts, enlisting a friend or family member as a virtual accountability partner offers a compromise, combining the flexibility of indepen-dent exercise with the motivational boost of social support.

In essence, low-impact workouts embody a philosophy of inclu-sivity and personalization, offering a spectrum of activities that cater to diverse needs and preferences. From the solitary wanderer relishing the meditative solitude of a walk to the social butterfly thriving in the communal energy of a yoga class, these exercises provide a foundation upon which individuals can build a lifestyle of sustained physical activity. Through thoughtful selection, integra-tion of variety and progression, and strategies to overcome barriers, low-impact workouts not only enhance physical health across all levels of fitness but also enrich the tapestry of daily life with the joy of movement.

4.4 THE ROLE OF FLEXIBILITY AND BALANCE IN AGING GRACEFULLY

In the tapestry of physical well-being, the threads of flexibility and balance are interwoven, essential for the fluidity and harmony of movement that define a life lived with vitality. The degradation of these physical attributes often accompanies the advancing years. Yet, their preservation is pivotal in maintaining autonomy and preventing the falls that frequently undermine the health of older adults. Flexibility, the capacity of muscles to elongate and allow for a full range of motion in the joints, diminishes with time as muscles naturally lose their elasticity. Balance, a complex coordination of muscular reactions, bone stability, and vestibular function, similarly faces decline, yet both can be significantly bolstered through deliberate practice.

Exercises that enhance flexibility often involve stretching routines that gently coax the muscles into greater lengths, promoting elasticity and reducing the stiffness that can restrict movement and contribute to discomfort and injury. Yoga, with its array of postures from the gentle forward fold to the expansive reach of the warrior poses, serves not only to stretch but to strengthen the muscles, supporting them in their quest for greater flexibility. This dual benefit underscores the value of yoga as a tool for maintaining and enhancing range of motion, making daily activities from bending to reach a shelf to looking over one's shoulder while driving more accessible and pain-free.

Balance training exercises, in contrast, focus on improving the body's ability to maintain its center of gravity amidst both static and dynamic conditions. Simple exercises like standing on one foot or walking heel-to-toe along a straight line can significantly improve balance by challenging the body to maintain stability. Tai chi, an ancient martial art known for its slow, deliberate movements and focus on breath control, is particularly effective in enhancing balance. Its sequences of movements, which flow smoothly from one to the next, challenge the body to adjust and stabilize continuously, strengthening the core muscles and improving proprioception, the body's sense of its position in space.

Integrating flexibility and balance exercises into daily routines can transform these practices from isolated workouts into integral components of everyday life. Stretching exercises, for instance, can be incorporated into morning routines, offering a gentle awakening for the body and preparing it for the day ahead. Similarly, balance exercises can be woven into activities such as brushing teeth or cooking, where one might practice standing on one leg for short periods. This seamless integration ensures consistent practice, a critical factor in maintaining and improving these physical attributes. Moreover, such practices encourage mindfulness and a deeper connection with one's body, fostering an awareness that becomes invaluable in preventing falls and injuries.

Embedding these exercises into the fabric of daily life does not necessitate significant alterations to one's schedule but rather a mindful adjustment to moments already present in the day. It invites a shift in perception, where every step and stretch becomes an opportunity to enhance well-being. The adoption of these practices, marked by regularity and intention, promises not only improved flexibility and balance but also a profound impact on overall health, contributing to a reduction in fall risk and an increase in the ability to perform daily activities with ease and confidence.

The pursuit of flexibility and balance, therefore, becomes not just an exercise in physical maintenance but a testament to the body's remarkable capacity for adaptation and renewal. It underscores the importance of holistic approaches to aging, where the focus extends beyond the mere prolongation of life to the enhancement of the quality of those years. Through dedicated practice, the aging body can retain, and even regain, the grace and agility that allow for an active, engaged existence.

Reflecting on my wellness journey, I've noticed a significant transformation in my priorities. Once, my workouts were dominated by a relentless pursuit of strength and endurance, with little regard for flexibility. However, as I ventured into my 50s, the emphasis naturally shifted towards flexibility, which surprisingly also led to an improvement in my overall strength. This shift highlights the critical importance of flexibility and balance as we age, showcasing their roles not just in maintaining grace but also in enhancing physical strength. Incorporating stretching and balance exercises into daily life has proven to be a cornerstone of maintaining physical health, ensuring each movement is both stable and fluid. This transition from focusing purely on physical attributes to embracing the mental and emotional facets of wellness underscores a holistic view of health, emphasizing the importance of a mindful, integrated approach as we navigate through the continuum of human well-being.

BIOHACKING YOUR WAY TO OPTIMAL HEALTH

In the labyrinth of wellness and longevity, red-light therapy emerges not as a mere speck of light but as a beacon, guiding through the shadows of conventional health practices into the luminescence of cellular rejuvenation. This method, while modern in its application, harks back to the dawn of consciousness when sunlight, in its full spectrum, served as the ultimate source of life and healing. Today, red-light therapy, a concentrated form of this primal energy, offers a key to unlocking health benefits that extend far beyond the visible.

5.1 RED-LIGHT THERAPY: SKIN HEALTH AND BEYOND

Understanding Red-Light Therapy

Red-light therapy, or low-level laser therapy (LLLT), operates on a simple premise: specific wavelengths of light, particularly in the red to near-infrared spectrum, penetrate the skin to various depths, stimulating cellular repair and rejuvenation without inflicting damage. The mitochondria, often dubbed the "powerhouses" of the cells, absorb this light, prompting a cascade of metabolic events that lead to an increase in cellular energy (ATP) production, reduction of oxidative stress, and enhanced DNA repair. These processes collectively not only bolster cell vitality but also fortify the body's defenses against the wear and tear of aging.

Benefits Beyond Skin Health

Red-light therapy's benefits transcend mere skin enhancement—its prowess in stimulating collagen production, smoothing out wrinkles, and accelerating wound healing is well recognized. However, its therapeutic reach delves deeper, targeting the body's musculoskeletal system with profound efficacy. Athletes and individuals grappling with chronic musculoskeletal ailments report significant relief under its radiant embrace, citing faster muscle recovery, alleviated joint pain, and a notable decrease in inflammation. This therapy shines not only in physical recovery but also in bolstering cognitive health. Rigorous studies have showcased a spectrum of cognitive improvements attributed to red-light therapy, including enhanced mood, sharper cognitive functions, and better sleep quality. These multifaceted benefits highlight red-light therapy's role as an indispensable component in the biohacking arsenal, championing not just superficial beauty but fostering an all-encompassing state of holistic well-being.

Initially, I harbored significant doubts about the efficacy of red-light therapy, struggling to grasp how exposure to red light could yield therapeutic benefits. Nonetheless, I remained open to further exploration, undeterred by my initial skepticism. Encouraged by many positive testimonials, including one from Dana White, I embarked on my own journey with this modality. Given the substantial investment required for red-light therapy beds, blankets, and wraps, I sought a more accessible entry point. Many tanning salons now offer red-light therapy beds, which provided me with an affordable and convenient option. For approximately $60, I secured a one-month membership and commenced my experiment. The initial sessions didn't produce any noticeable effects beyond a mild warmth. However, by the second week, I started experiencing a reduction in stiffness, which indirectly boosted my energy levels by alleviating the constant discomfort of inflammation. As the end of my membership approached, the improvements were undeniable, compelling me to invest in a red-light therapy blanket wrap akin to a sleeping bag. This device has since become an integral component of my and my wife's wellness regimen, underscoring the transformative power of red-light therapy in our pursuit of health and vitality.

How to Safely Use Red-Light Therapy

Navigating red-light therapy involves balancing efficacy and safety, a harmony achieved through the judicious choice between at-home devices and professional treatments. For those seeking convenience, at-home devices offer a practical solution, enabling daily sessions that fit seamlessly into personal routines. Yet, selecting these devices demands scrutiny, focusing on parameters such as wavelength, irradiance, and treatment area coverage to ensure therapeutic effectiveness. On the other end of the spectrum, professional treatments, administered in clinical settings, provide the advantage of higher-powered devices and tailored treatment protocols, overseen by practitioners versed in the nuances of light therapy. Regardless of the setting, adherence to recommended durations and frequencies of treatment is paramount to avoid potential side effects, ensuring a safe journey towards enhanced health.

Evidence-Based Review

The tapestry of research surrounding red-light therapy weaves a compelling narrative of its efficacy. A meta-analysis in the *Journal of Photochemistry and Photobiology* synthesizes data from multiple studies, highlighting significant improvements in skin complexion, collagen density, and wound healing among participants. In the realm of muscle recovery, research published in the *Journal of Athletic Training* reveals a marked reduction in muscle soreness and inflammation post-exercise, underscoring the therapy's role in enhancing athletic performance. Cognitive benefits, too, find grounding in science, with a study in the *Journal of Neuroscience* reporting improved memory and mood among subjects exposed to near-infrared light. These varied findings converge on a singular point: red-light therapy, when applied with precision and care, holds the key to unlocking a spectrum of health benefits, heralding a new dawn in the quest for longevity.

Visual Element: Red-Light Therapy Device Comparison Chart

A meticulously crafted infographic titled "Choosing the Right Red-Light Therapy Device" offers a visual guide for navigating the market of at-home devices. This chart details critical specifications —wavelengths, power output, FDA approval status, and recommended usage times—across various popular models. It provides a clear, comparative analysis that empowers readers to make informed choices based on their specific health goals and budgetary constraints.

In the embrace of red-light therapy, we find a convergence of ancient wisdom and modern science. This union illuminates a path towards enhanced health and longevity. Through a nuanced understanding of its mechanisms, a broad appreciation of its benefits, and a mindful approach to its application, this therapeutic light stands as a testament to the enduring quest for wellness, offering a beacon of hope and healing in the complex landscape of biohacking.

5.2 THE BENEFITS OF COLD EXPOSURE: MYTH VS. REALITY

Cold exposure, a term that encapsulates the deliberate act of subjecting the body to low temperatures, has roots that burrow deep into the annals of human evolution. This practice, far from being a mere test of endurance, unfolds on the cellular stage, where the cold triggers a symphony of physiological responses designed to fortify health. At the core of this adaptive process lies thermogenesis, the body's mechanism for generating heat. Two forms, shivering and non-shivering thermogenesis, play pivotal roles. Shivering thermogenesis involves rapid muscle contractions, a primitive yet effective method of heat production. More intriguing, however, is non-shivering thermogenesis, where brown adipose tissue (BAT) metabolizes fat into heat, offering a metabolic advantage that extends beyond mere survival to embrace enhanced metabolic efficiency and weight regulation.

In exploring cold exposure modalities, three distinct practices emerge cold showers, ice baths, and winter swimming. Each method, varying in intensity and duration, caters to different thresholds of tolerance and health objectives. Cold showers, the most accessible of the trio, serve as an invigorating entry point, accelerating the heart rate and enhancing blood circulation. This acute cardiovascular response, coupled with the shower's ability to refine mood through the release of endorphins, positions it as a dual-purpose tool for physiological and psychological uplift. Ice baths, a notch higher on the intensity scale, immerse the body in near-freezing water, a practice lauded by athletes for its profound impact on muscle recovery and inflammation reduction. The abrupt and substantial drop in temperature encountered in an ice bath pushes the body to adapt, strengthening the cardiovascular system and enhancing immune function. Winter swimming, the most extreme in terms of exposure and environmental challenge, combines the benefits of cold immersion with the physical demands of swimming, offering a potent stimulus for cardiovascular health, metabolic rate enhancement, and immunity boosting.

Despite the growing body of evidence supporting the health benefits of cold exposure, myths and misconceptions cloud its application. Fears of hypothermia and immune suppression, while valid in contexts of prolonged, unprotected exposure to extreme cold, do not typically apply to controlled cold exposure practices. On the contrary, research delineates how regular, moderated cold exposure can amplify the immune response, increasing the count of white blood cells and circulating levels of immune-boosting proteins. The myth that cold exposure invariably leads to increased susceptibility to infections thus unravels, revealing a narrative of resilience and enhanced defense mechanisms. Another common misconception posits that cold exposure is inherently detrimental to cardiovascular health. While individuals with pre-existing heart conditions should proceed with caution, for the healthy population, cold exposure has been shown to fortify cardiovascular function by improving vascular elasticity and reducing inflammation, a testament to the body's remarkable capacity not only to endure but thrive under the stimulus of cold.

For those intrigued by the potential of cold exposure to elevate health, a practical guide to incorporation offers a pathway to safely harness this elemental force. The initiation into cold exposure best begins with gradual adaptation, starting with brief, lukewarm showers that progressively shift to cooler temperatures. This step-wise approach allows the body to acclimate to the cold, minimizing shock and discomfort. As comfort with the cold increases, the duration of exposure can extend, and the temperature can decrease, steering towards the eventual integration of ice baths or winter swimming into the wellness regimen. Throughout this process, mindfulness of the body's signals remains paramount; sensations of undue stress or discomfort serve as cues to moderate the intensity or duration of exposure. Additionally, the practice of warming up post-exposure, whether through physical activity or a warm environment, ensures a balanced recovery, preventing undue thermal stress.

In the realm of cold exposure, the delineation between myth and reality unfolds as a narrative of empowerment, where informed practice dispels fear, and the body's innate adaptability shines. Through the strategic application of cold showers, ice baths, and winter swimming, individuals can tap into a wellspring of health benefits, from metabolic enhancement to immune fortification. This journey, marked not by the pursuit of extremity but by the embrace of moderation and mindfulness, reveals the transformative potential of cold exposure, a testament to the body's profound capacity for resilience and renewal.

Integrating cold exposure into my daily routine was a brutal challenge. The mere thought of deliberately subjecting myself to cold regularly seemed almost insane. Recalling my college days, I remembered the numerous occasions when our team trainer would prescribe an ice bath for various strains or sprains incurred during practice. I would concoct every conceivable excuse to evade this chilly remedy, often without success. However, during my research, the benefits of cold exposure emerged as consistently as the use of turmeric, supported by a plethora of studies showcasing significant positive outcomes across multiple health aspects. With some reluctance, I started with ice-cold showers as a gentle introduction to cold exposure. Though these sessions are recommended to last between 3 to 6 minutes, my initial attempts barely reached 60 to 90 seconds. In contrast, my wife easily surpassed the 4-minute mark from the start, sometimes extending her exposure to 10 minutes. Obviously, she is much tougher than me. Despite my gradual progress toward the 4-minute goal, the impact of cold exposure on my overall energy and focus, particularly in the mornings, has been unmistakably profound.

5.3 ELEVATING HEALTH WITH HYDROGEN WATER

Intriguing developments in the realm of wellness spotlight hydrogen water, a seemingly simple concoction that veils profound implications for human health beneath its effervescent surface. This variant of water, saturated with molecular hydrogen, invites a closer examination of its role as a potent antioxidant. The premise that underpins the enthusiasm for hydrogen-rich water hinges on the molecule's ability to permeate the body's cellular defenses, offering protection against the oxidative stress that accelerates the aging process and predisposes to chronic diseases.

At the heart of hydrogen water's appeal is its purported capacity to act as an antioxidant. The science elucidates how molecular hydrogen, due to its diminutive size and neutral charge, diffuses with remarkable ease across cellular membranes, engaging rogue free radicals and neutralizing them without the collateral damage typical of more indiscriminate antioxidants. This selective antioxidant activity posits hydrogen water as a guardian against oxidative damage, with the potential to mitigate inflammation, slow cellular aging, and bolster metabolic health.

Scrutiny of the health claims surrounding hydrogen water reveals a landscape marked by both promising research and areas awaiting further exploration. Studies, albeit preliminary, illuminate the beneficial effects of hydrogen-enriched water on markers of inflammation and oxidative stress. For instance, research in sports science indicates that athletes consuming hydrogen water exhibit a marked reduction in lactic acid buildup post-exercise, a metric of reduced oxidative stress and improved recovery times. Similarly, investigations into metabolic syndrome, a constellation of conditions that heightens the risk of heart disease, stroke, and diabetes, suggest that hydrogen water may improve lipid profiles and glucose metabolism, pointing towards its potential role in metabolic health. Nevertheless, the scientific community maintains a stance of cautious optimism, advocating for more rigorous, large-scale studies to substantiate these findings and fully unveil the spectrum of hydrogen water's health benefits.

Incorporating hydrogen water into one's daily regimen unfolds as an exercise in simplicity and mindfulness. The market offers a range of options for introducing molecular hydrogen into drinking water, from ready-to-drink bottles to tablets that dissolve in water, releasing hydrogen gas. For those seeking a more integrated approach, hydrogen water generators provide a steady supply, ensuring that the benefits of hydrogen-rich water are but a glass away. The frequency and timing of consumption hinge on personal preferences and goals; however, integrating a glass of hydrogen water in the morning routine or as a post-exercise replenishment can serve as a practical starting point. Mindful consumption, attuned to the body's responses, allows individuals to adjust their intake of hydrogen water, aligning it with their specific health objectives and lifestyle.

Incorporating hydrogen water into my daily wellness routine significantly improved my health and vitality. The process of adding this element to my daily habits was surprisingly easy and meshed well with my existing routines. In a brief period of steady consumption, I experienced a noticeable boost in energy— a change that was both quick and profound. This increase in energy not only enhanced my physical health but also sharpened my mental clarity and bolstered my capacity to face daily tasks. The simplicity of incorporating hydrogen water into one's daily life, combined with swift and positive outcomes, highlights its effectiveness as a powerful means to achieve peak health and longevity. I prefer a portable, rechargeable hydrogen water bottle, capable of producing 990 ppm, offering flexibility at home, work, during exercise, or while on the move. With an extensive selection of quality devices available online, adopting this impressive health hack into your routine is both straightforward and achievable.

5.4 GROUNDING: CONNECTING WITH THE EARTH'S ENERGY

In the domain of biohacking, an ancient practice often overlooked, whispers of healing and connection. Grounding, or earthing, refers to direct contact with the earth's surface. This simple yet profound communion channels the planet's electrons into the body. This interaction, elemental in its essence, taps into the earth's inherent electrical fields, a vast reservoir of natural energy that, when engaged, promises to recalibrate and rejuvenate the body's own electrical circuitry.

The inquiry into grounding's efficacy reveals a compelling array of potential health benefits, a spectrum that spans from the reduction of inflammation to the enhancement of sleep quality. The premise hinges on the earth's surface being laden with free electrons, potent in their antioxidative capacity. These electrons, upon contact, are thought to neutralize free radicals within the body, those rogue agents of inflammation and cellular damage. Empirical evidence lends weight to this theory, with studies indicating marked decreases in blood markers of inflammation among participants who engaged in regular grounding practices. Sleep, too, falls under grounding's gentle sway, with anecdotal and research-backed accounts highlighting improvements in both duration and quality. Pain reduction, particularly chronic pain associated with conditions like fibromyalgia, has also been reported, offering a beacon of relief for those trapped in the grip of discomfort.

Adopting grounding into daily routines emerges not as a Herculean feat but as an accessible venture that transcends urban constraints and the intricacies of modern living. The simplest method involves barefoot walks on grass, soil, or sand, an act that fosters connection not only with the earth but with the environment at large. For individuals inhabiting urban landscapes, where direct contact with the earth might prove elusive, grounding mats and sheets present an alternative, simulating the electrical exchange between the body and the ground. These devices, designed for use during sleep or sedentary activities, extend grounding's reach into the realms of home and office, ensuring continuous access to its restorative potential. Beyond these interventions, cultivating mindfulness around the practice amplifies its benefits, turning moments of grounding into opportunities for reflection and presence.

Narratives of transformation abound, painting vivid portraits of lives touched and altered by grounding. One such account comes from a middle-aged man grappling with the insidious creep of insomnia and the pervasive fog of chronic fatigue. His introduction to grounding, initially met with skepticism, evolved into a cornerstone of his wellness regimen, with nightly practices of sleeping on a grounding mat ushering in deeper rest and a resurgence of vitality. Another story unfolds from a woman beset by the relentless ache of arthritis, her days colored by pain and limitation. Through regular, barefoot walks in her garden, she discovered not only a gradual easing of discomfort but a renewed sense of connection with the natural world, a dual gift of relief and reawakening.

These stories, each unique in its contours, converge on a singular theme: grounding's capacity to mend and to soothe, to reconnect the individual with the rhythms of the earth. They serve as testaments to the practice's simplicity and its profound impact, underscoring the potential that lies in reaching down and touching the ground, in bridging the gap between the human body and the earth's vast, healing energy.

In reflection, this exploration of grounding, nestled within the broader context of biohacking and wellness, illuminates a path that is both ancient and urgently relevant. It invites a reevaluation of our relationship with the natural world, urging a return to simplicity in our quest for health. Grounding, with its roots deep in the primal soil of human experience, offers a method for enhancing physical well-being and a paradigm for living that recognizes the interconnectedness of body, earth, and spirit. As we advance into the subsequent chapters, this theme of connection—between ourselves, our environment, and our health—continues to unfurl, guiding us toward a holistic understanding of wellness that encompasses not only the body and mind but also the soul and the soil underfoot.

NOURISHING LONGEVITY FROM THE WORLD'S BLUE ZONES

A thread, when followed back to its origin, often leads to a tapestry of interconnected wisdom and tradition. Such is the case with the dietary habits found in the world's Blue Zones—regions known for their extraordinary lifespans and minimal incidence of chronic diseases. These pockets of longevity, scattered across the globe, offer not just clues but tangible evidence of how diet influences health and lifespan. In examining these dietary patterns, one finds a commonality that transcends geographical and cultural boundaries, pointing toward a universal blueprint for health.

6.1 DIETARY SECRETS FROM THE BLUE ZONES

Identifying the Blue Zones

Researchers, after meticulous study, pinpointed five regions: Okinawa (Japan), Sardinia (Italy), Nicoya (Costa Rica), Icaria (Greece), and Loma Linda (California, USA), as the epicenters of longevity. These Blue Zones, so named for the azure ink used to circle them on a researcher's map, emerged from a quest to understand the secrets behind their residents' remarkable lifespans. It's a quest that, much like sifting through the layers of an archaeological dig, reveals the foundations of health and longevity built upon diet, lifestyle, and community.

Key Dietary Patterns

A closer look at the diets in these regions uncovers a pattern that is as simple in composition as profound in its impact. Predominantly plant-based, these diets spotlight legumes, whole grains, vegetables, fruits, nuts, and seeds as staples. For instance, Olive oil in Sardinia and Icaria emerges not just as a culinary preference but as a cornerstone of health, its monounsaturated fats combating inflammation and heart disease. In Okinawa, sweet potatoes, rich in beta-carotene and fiber, form the dietary bedrock, supporting metabolic health and longevity. Moderate consumption of alcohol, particularly red wine in Sardinia and Icaria, introduces antioxidants like resveratrol, which protect against heart disease. Fasting rituals, whether through the Adventist Sabbath in Loma Linda or the Orthodox Christian practices in Icaria, introduce periods of caloric restriction, which research links to improved metabolic health and increased lifespan.

Adapting Blue Zone Diets to Modern Living

Translating these dietary principles into the rhythm of contemporary life might seem a Sisyphean task in a world awash with processed foods and fast-paced living. Yet, integrating Blue Zone-inspired habits need not be an overhaul but a series of purposeful adjustments. Incorporating a "meatless Monday," substituting olive oil for butter, snacking on nuts instead of processed foods, or dedicating a day to fasting can bridge centuries-old wisdom with modern dietary practices. These changes, modest yet impactful, weave the longevity practices of the Blue Zones into the fabric of daily life, making health and longevity accessible to all.

Case Studies

Visual Element: Blue Zones Dietary Pyramid Infographic

An infographic, "The Blue Zones Dietary Pyramid," distills the essence of Blue Zone diets into a visual guide. At its base, the pyramid is broad with vegetables, fruits, whole grains, and legumes, illustrating their foundational role. Ascending the pyramid, fish and lean meats appear in moderation, with red meat and processed foods at the pinnacle, indicating their limited consumption. This visual tool not only simplifies the dietary habits that underscore longevity in the Blue Zones but also serves as a daily reference for meal planning and grocery shopping, making the principles of longevity an integral part of dietary choices.

In drawing inspiration from the Blue Zones, one finds not just a diet but a philosophy of eating that celebrates the richness of the earth's bounty, the joy of shared meals, and the profound impact of simple, whole foods on health and longevity. These regions, with their diverse cultures and traditions, converge on a universal truth: that the keys to a long, vibrant life are often found not in the complexity of modern dietary regimes but in the simplicity and wisdom of the past.

6.2 COMMUNITY AND SOCIAL CONNECTIONS: LEARNING FROM OKINAWA

In the heart of Okinawa, an island draped in the vibrancy of age-old traditions and the wisdom of its elders, lies a profound understanding of social cohesion's intrinsic value to health and longevity. This societal fabric, meticulously woven with threads of camaraderie, support, and shared purpose, presents a compelling tableau of how deep-rooted connections can significantly enhance one's lifespan and quality of life. The Okinawan concept of "moai," a term that encapsulates the essence of forming lifelong support networks, embodies a practice where groups of individuals commit to each other's well-being, creating a formidable bastion against the isolating tendencies of modern living.

The genesis of a "moai" finds its roots in the economic needs of ancient Okinawan communities, where farmers and fishermen banded together to share resources and labor. However, this pragmatic arrangement blossomed into a profound societal bond, transcending material assistance to offer emotional support, companionship, and collective wisdom. These circles of friends navigate life's vicissitudes together, celebrating joys, shouldering burdens, and providing a sense of belonging that nourishes both the mind and body. Through the lens of "moai," the intertwining of social ties with longevity emerges not as a serendipitous correlation but as a causal nexus, where robust social networks directly contribute to enhanced health outcomes.

Strategies for fostering such connections in societies increasingly characterized by fragmentation and solitude draw inspiration from the Okinawan example. The initiation of community groups centered around shared interests or stages of life serves as a foundational step, inviting individuals to partake in collective activities that foster mutual understanding and support. From book clubs and gardening cohorts to walking groups and volunteer organizations, these assemblies function as modern-day "moais," providing platforms for regular interaction and the formation of meaningful relationships. Furthermore, the integration of technology, while often criticized for its role in social isolation, presents an opportunity to bridge distances and cultivate virtual communities where geographical constraints might otherwise preclude connection.

The repercussions of these social integrations on mental and physical health are profound, illuminated by a growing body of research that underscores the protective effects of strong social networks. Studies reveal a marked reduction in mortality risk among individuals with dense social connections, a phenomenon attributed to the stress-buffering effect of emotional support and the positive influence of social norms on health behaviors. The alleviation of loneliness, a condition linked with elevated risks of heart disease and mental decline, further exemplifies the health dividends of social integration. In Okinawa, where elder care is often a communal responsibility, the incidence of depression and cognitive disorders among seniors remains notably low, a testament to the beneficial effects of social engagement on mental health.

In dissecting the mechanisms through which social connections wield their influence on health, the interplay between psychological well-being and physiological function becomes apparent. Social bonds, characterized by trust, empathy, and mutual aid, engender a sense of security and self-worth that mitigates stress and its corrosive effects on the body. The consequent reduction in stress hormones, such as cortisol, coupled with the promotion of positive affective states, enhances immune function and reduces inflammation, fortifying the body against various age-related ailments. Moreover, the adoption of healthful behaviors within social groups—from dietary habits to physical activity—fosters a culture of wellness that propels individuals toward healthier lifestyles, further entrenching the link between social connections and longevity.

In Okinawa, the seamless blend of social integration with daily life offers a blueprint for countering the malaise of isolation that pervades much of the modern world. The cultivation of "moai"-like networks, whether through deliberate community-building efforts or the leveraging of digital platforms to sustain connections, underscores the actionable nature of this longevity secret. It is a call to action for societies grappling with the challenges of aging populations and rising rates of loneliness, highlighting the necessity of fostering environments where social ties can flourish.

Through the prism of Okinawan culture, the critical role of community and social connections in nurturing health and extending life unfurls with clarity and urgency. This understanding, rooted in centuries of lived experience, beckons a reevaluation of societal priorities, placing the nurturing of human connections at the forefront of public health initiatives. It is a recognition that the journey toward a fuller, longer life is one best traveled with companions in the spirit of "moai," where the collective pursuit of well-being illuminates the path to longevity.

6.3 STRESS MANAGEMENT TECHNIQUES FROM THE WORLD'S OLDEST PEOPLE

In the pursuit of longevity, the management of stress is not merely a practice but a necessity, woven into the fabric of daily life by those who have surpassed the century mark. These individuals residing in regions celebrated for their remarkable lifespans approach stress not as an inevitable burden but as a variable that can be modified and controlled through lifestyle, community engagement, and a perspective prioritizing tranquility and balance. Within these practices and outlooks, one can find keys to mitigating the modern era's relentless stressors.

Centenarians, through the rhythm of their routines, demonstrate a profound alignment with the natural cadence of life, a harmony that inherently dispels the chaos of stress. Daily activities, whether tending to a garden, preparing meals from scratch, or engaging in gentle physical activity, are not rushed but embraced with mindfulness, allowing for a presence of mind that keeps stress at bay. Moreover, involvement in community activities serves as a source of personal fulfillment and a buffer against the solitude that can amplify stress. The perspective these elders hold, viewing life's challenges not as insurmountable obstacles but as transient phases, further cements their resilience against stress. This outlook, cultivated over decades, fosters a sense of acceptance and adaptability, qualities that are indispensable in managing life's unpredictable nature.

The arsenal of stress-reduction techniques employed by these longevity champions includes practices steeped in tradition yet timeless in their efficacy. Meditation, a cornerstone of many cultures known for their longevity, offers a refuge from the mental clutter that fuels stress. This practice, varying from the focused attention on breath in zazen to the recitation of mantras in transcendental meditation, cultivates a state of mental clarity and calm that counteracts the physiological responses to stress. Nap rituals, embraced in regions such as the Mediterranean, underscore the recognition of rest as a fundamental pillar of health, providing the body with a pause that resets the stress response. Community festivals, a staple in the social calendar of many Blue Zones, foster a sense of belonging and joy, elevating communal well-being and diluting individual stress through shared experiences of celebration and connection.

Adapting these time-honored strategies to the pressures of contemporary life might appear daunting, yet it is within reach through intentional adjustments to daily routines. Integrating moments of meditation into the morning or evening can anchor the day with a sense of calm, setting a tone that helps navigate stress with grace.

Embracing short naps or periods of rest, especially during times of heightened stress, can provide the mental and physical respite needed to maintain balance. Participation in community events or creating such gatherings in one's own circle can rekindle the sense of connection and joy that mitigates stress and enriches life with purpose and belonging.

The relationship between stress and longevity is illuminated by a growing body of research that underscores the harmful effects of chronic stress on the aging process. Elevated cortisol levels, a hallmark of the stress response, have been linked to accelerated cellular aging, manifesting in telomere shortening and increased inflammation—factors that contribute to the onset of age-related diseases. The practices of centenarians, rooted in routines that diffuse stress, communal activities that foster connection, and a perspective that embraces life's ebb and flow, naturally counteract these biological responses to stress. By reducing cortisol levels, enhancing immune function, and promoting a state of mental well-being, these practices offer a blueprint for not only navigating but thriving amidst life's inherent stressors.

In essence, the techniques for managing stress, exemplified by the world's oldest people, embody a holistic approach to well-being that transcends the absence of disease. It is an approach that integrates the physical, mental, and social dimensions of health, offering a comprehensive strategy for extending not only the length of life but the quality of those years. Through the adaptation of these practices —mindfulness in daily activities, traditional stress-reduction techniques, and the cultivation of a resilient perspective—one can navigate the modern world's complexities with a sense of tranquility and balance that is the hallmark of true longevity.

6.4 PHYSICAL ACTIVITY AS A WAY OF LIFE IN LONGEVITY CULTURES

In cultures distinguished by unparalleled longevity, the fabric of daily existence is interwoven with the threads of moderate, continuous physical activity. This seamless melding of movement with the rhythm of life stands in stark contrast to the segmented nature of exercise in the modern Western paradigm, where physical activity often exists in discrete blocks of time carved out from the day's obligations. For inhabitants of longevity cultures, movement is not an interruption to daily life but an integral aspect of it, a natural expression of living that maintains physical vitality well into the later years.

Gardening, an almost universal practice among these cultures, serves not merely as a means to nourish the body with fresh produce but as a form of exercise that engages the whole body. The acts of bending, lifting, digging, and walking across the garden plot comprise a comprehensive physical workout that enhances flexibility, strength, and cardiovascular health. Moreover, the connection to the earth and the cycle of life that gardening fosters contributes to mental well-being, illustrating the holistic benefits of this form of natural movement.

Walking, another cornerstone of activity in longevity cultures, is less about the deliberate pursuit of exercise and more about an intrinsic aspect of daily routines. Whether it's walking to the local market, visiting neighbors, or simply taking a leisurely stroll through the community, this form of movement integrates cardiovascular exercise into the day without the need for special equipment or designated time. The benefits extend beyond the physical, fostering social interactions and a deep connection with one's environment, further enhancing the quality of life.

Traditional crafts, too, play a role in the physical culture of these communities. Activities such as weaving, pottery, and woodworking are not only expressions of cultural heritage but also involve sustained, repetitive motions that build dexterity, fine motor skills, and even endurance. Engaging in these crafts represents a form of physical activity that is mentally engaging and emotionally satisfying, contributing to a well-rounded, active lifestyle.

The modern challenge lies in translating these integrated, natural movement principles into a lifestyle increasingly characterized by sedentary habits. The key lies in creating opportunities for movement that align with the flow of daily life rather than existing outside of it. Simple adjustments, such as choosing stairs over elevators, parking further away from destinations to encourage walking, or incorporating standing desks into work environments, can significantly increase daily physical activity levels. Cultivating hobbies that involve physical movement, such as gardening or cycling, offers a dual benefit of exercise and personal enjoyment, seamlessly blending the concept of movement with the art of living.

Inspiration flows from the stories of centenarians who maintain remarkable levels of activity, their lifestyles a testament to the enduring capacity of the human body. One such individual, at the age of 102, continues to tend her vegetable garden daily, a ritual that sustains her both physically and spiritually. Another, aged 100, walks two miles every morning, a practice he credits not only with his longevity but with his mental clarity and zest for life. These narratives underscore the foundational belief that movement is life and that sustaining physical activity is vital to sustaining life itself.

As this exploration of movement in longevity cultures concludes, the core principles emerge with clarity. The integration of moderate, continuous physical activity into the fabric of daily life, the embrace of natural forms of exercise such as gardening, walking, and traditional crafts, and the inspiration drawn from individuals who embody these practices offer a blueprint for a life characterized by vitality and longevity. This approach, rooted in the wisdom of cultures that have nurtured long, healthy lives through centuries, invites a reimagining of physical activity not as a chore but as a joyous expression of living. It beckons a shift towards lifestyles that honor the innate human need for movement, weaving the threads of activity into the tapestry of daily existence.

As we transition from the exploration of physical activity to the realms of mental and emotional well-being, these principles of movement serve not only as a foundation for physical health but as a metaphor for the dynamic, integrated approach to wellness that defines the journey toward optimal health. This holistic perspective, recognizing the interplay between physical activity, mental clarity, and emotional resilience, guides us toward a comprehensive understanding of well-being that transcends the boundaries of age and culture, leading us into the next chapter of our exploration.

MINDFULNESS AND MEDITATION: PATHWAYS TO LONGEVITY

In a world awash with the constant hum of activity, the ancient practices of meditation and mindfulness stand as quiet sentinels, guardians of tranquility and longevity. These practices, steeped in centuries of tradition, offer a counterpoint to the frenetic pace of modern life, inviting a reflective pause that rejuvenates both mind and body. At their core, meditation and mindfulness embody a profound simplicity: the act of being present, fully and completely, in the moment. Yet, within this simplicity lies a complexity of benefits that extend far beyond the immediate calm they provide, weaving into the very fabric of our being and potentially extending our lifespan.

7.1 THE SCIENCE OF MEDITATION AND MINDFULNESS IN LONGEVITY

Overview of Meditation Practices

Meditation, with its diverse forms, from the focused tranquility of Zen to the loving-kindness (Metta) meditation, offers a spectrum of pathways to inner peace. Each style possesses its unique flavor, catering to varied preferences and objectives, yet all share the common goal of silencing the chatter of the mind to uncover the serene awareness beneath. Vipassana, for example, emphasizes observation of the breath or bodily sensations as a means to transcend thought, fostering a state of detached awareness. Conversely, transcendental meditation uses a mantra as a focal point to guide the practitioner into deeper levels of consciousness.

Mindfulness and Its Impact on Aging

Mindfulness, a practice deeply intertwined with meditation, centers on maintaining a moment-by-moment awareness of our thoughts, feelings, bodily sensations, and the surrounding environment. This attentiveness cultivates a profound connection to the present, enabling individuals to engage fully with life as it unfolds. The implications of mindfulness for aging are profound, with research suggesting that consistent practice can mitigate stress, bolster cognitive function, and enhance emotional well-being. A study published in the journal *Psychosomatic Medicine* revealed that mindfulness meditation is associated with decreased levels of the stress hormone cortisol, which has been implicated in accelerated aging and cognitive decline.

Implementing a Consistent Meditation Routine

For those new to meditation, the prospect of integrating this practice into daily life might seem daunting. A practical approach involves starting small, with just a few minutes each day, and gradually increasing the duration as comfort with the practice grows. Morning, a time of natural quiet, offers an ideal backdrop for meditation, setting a foundation of calm for the day ahead. Alternatively, evening sessions can serve as a soothing transition to rest, aiding in the release of the day's tensions. Digital platforms and apps provide guided sessions that ease beginners into the practice, offering a structured path toward developing a consistent routine.

Research and Case Studies

The tangible benefits of meditation and mindfulness for longevity are underscored by a growing body of scientific research. A landmark study in the *Journal of Neuroscience* demonstrated that regular meditation not only reduces stress but can also lead to structural changes in the brain, including increased grey matter density in areas associated with memory, empathy, and stress regulation. Further, a paper in the *American Journal of Geriatric Psychiatry* found that participants who practiced mindfulness showed signs of reduced cellular aging, as evidenced by the maintenance of telomere length, critical indicators of cellular longevity.

Visual Element: Daily Meditation Tracker

A visually engaging Daily Meditation Tracker, formatted as an interactive PDF, encourages practitioners to monitor their progress. This tracker, designed with simplicity in mind, allows users to log their daily practice, noting the duration, style of meditation, and any reflections or insights that arise. By providing a tangible record of their journey, individuals can witness the evolution of their practice over time, fostering a sense of accomplishment and deepening their commitment to this life-enhancing habit.

In the realm of wellness and longevity, meditation and mindfulness emerge not as mere ancillary practices but as central pillars supporting a life of vitality and extended healthspan. Through the serenity of meditation and the presence of mindfulness, individuals can access a wellspring of inner peace, resilience, and cognitive clarity, counteracting the stresses that age both mind and body. This chapter, dedicated to unraveling the intricate tapestry of benefits these practices offer, invites readers to explore the serene depths of their own consciousness, discovering therein the keys to a longer, more fulfilling existence.

7.2 YOGA AND TAI CHI: PHYSICAL BENEFITS AND BEYOND

In the tapestry of mind-body practices, yoga, and Tai Chi emerge as threads of ancient wisdom, meticulously woven through the fabric of contemporary wellness narratives. These disciplines, while distinct in their origins and methodologies, converge in their holistic approach to health, advocating for a seamless union of physical poise, mental tranquility, and emotional equilibrium. This section unravels the multifaceted dimensions of yoga and Tai Chi, elucidating their roles not merely as exercises but as profound avenues for enhancing life quality across the lifespan.

Yoga, a practice with roots burrowed deep in the fertile grounds of ancient Indian philosophy, transcends the confines of mere physical activity to embody a comprehensive lifestyle practice. At its essence, yoga harmonizes flexibility, strength, and mental clarity through a series of postures (asanas), breathing techniques (pranayama), and meditation (dhyana). Each asana, meticulously designed to align and strengthen the body, also serves as a conduit for focusing the mind, cultivating an attentive awareness that bridges the physical and the ethereal realms of existence. The adaptability of yoga allows individuals of all ages to tailor practices to their unique physical conditions and wellness goals, from gentle restorative sequences to more dynamic vinyasa flows, ensuring accessibility and sustainability of practice over time.

Tai Chi, often described as meditation in motion, originates from ancient Chinese martial arts, embodying principles of balance, fluidity, and grace. This gentle exercise, characterized by slow, deliberate movements synchronized with deep, rhythmic breathing, engages the practitioner in a flowing dance that mirrors the natural movements of life. Tai Chi's emphasis on weight shifting enhances balance and coordination, reducing the risk of falls, while its meditative aspects lower stress and promote a serene state of mind. The cardiovascular benefits, stemming from its moderate aerobic intensity, further underscore Tai Chi's efficacy as a holistic exercise modality suitable for individuals navigating the nuances of aging.

Incorporating yoga and Tai Chi into the relentless pace of modern life might appear as a daunting endeavor, yet the integration of these practices into daily routines unfolds with surprising fluidity. Initiating or concluding the day with a short yoga sequence can anchor the body in strength and the mind in clarity, preparing one for the challenges ahead or facilitating a transition into restful repose. Similarly, carving out moments for Tai Chi, perhaps during a lunch break or in the tranquility of an early evening, can serve as a rejuvenating pause, a respite amidst the day's tumult. For those constrained by schedules that defy the conventional, digital platforms offer guided sessions that bring the essence of these practices into any space, any time, democratizing access to these ancient wellness modalities.

The effectiveness of yoga and Tai Chi extends beyond anecdotal evidence, finding robust support in the annals of scientific research. A myriad of studies elucidates the impact of regular yoga practice on physical health, highlighting improvements in flexibility, muscle strength, and posture. Research in the *American Journal of Preventive Medicine* delineates yoga's role in mitigating chronic pain, particularly lower back pain, fostering an enhanced range of motion and functional mobility. Tai Chi, in its graceful complexity, offers similar benefits, with studies indicating significant reductions in stress, anxiety, and depression. The *Journal of the American Heart*

*Association*presents findings that underscore Tai Chi's positive effects on cardiovascular health, revealing improved blood pressure and lipid profiles among practitioners.

This exploration of yoga and Tai Chi, set against the backdrop of a world in dire need of balance and tranquility, illuminates these practices as beacons of holistic health. They stand not merely as physical exercises but as profound spiritual journeys that nurture the body, calm the mind, and soothe the soul. Through the deliberate movements of Tai Chi and the mindful postures of yoga, individuals find a path to wellness that transcends the boundaries of age and physical capability, embracing a journey toward a life of harmony, vitality, and longevity.

7.3 BIOFEEDBACK AND NEUROFEEDBACK FOR EMOTIONAL REGULATION

In the realm of technological advancements tailored to augment human health, biofeedback emerges as a beacon, illuminating the path to mastery over the often elusive internal processes that dictate well-being. This technique, grounded in the principles of operant conditioning, equips individuals with the ability to modulate physiological functions that are typically considered automatic, such as heart rate, muscle tension, and skin temperature, through real-time feedback. The essence of biofeedback lies in its empowering premise: by making the invisible visible, it grants individuals the agency to influence their health outcomes directly.

Simultaneously, neurofeedback, a specialized branch of biofeedback, focuses its lens on the electrical activity of the brain, offering a window into the neural symphonies that underlie cognitive functions and emotional states. This method holds the promise of optimizing brain performance, providing a non-invasive conduit to alleviate a spectrum of neurological and psychological challenges.

At its core, neurofeedback fosters an environment where the brain can learn to modulate its activity towards more balanced and efficient patterns, enhancing focus, reducing anxiety, and bolstering cognitive function.

The convergence of biofeedback and neurofeedback within the therapeutic landscape presents not only a frontier of mental health intervention but also a testament to the capacity for human innovation in the pursuit of wellness. Access to these therapies unfolds across a spectrum of avenues, from clinical settings where practitioners guide individuals through tailored protocols to the burgeoning market of home-use devices designed to bring the power of biofeedback and neurofeedback into the daily lives of users. The democratization of access to these technologies, however, is not without its challenges. The cost of professional-grade equipment and therapy sessions may pose barriers, yet the emergence of consumer devices offers a bridge, making the benefits of these practices more widely attainable.

The narratives of transformation that accompany biofeedback and neurofeedback therapies are as varied as they are profound. One account details the experience of a veteran grappling with post-traumatic stress disorder (PTSD), for whom traditional treatments had fallen short. Through neurofeedback, this individual learned to modulate their brain's response to stress triggers, gradually reducing the frequency and intensity of PTSD episodes and reclaiming a sense of calm that had seemed permanently out of reach. Another story unfolds from a student burdened by debilitating anxiety and concentration difficulties, challenges that had erected formidable barriers to academic and personal growth. Biofeedback sessions, focusing on heart rate variability, provided the tools to navigate anxiety with newfound control, leading to significant improvements in academic performance and overall quality of life.

These testimonials underscore the transformative potential of biofeedback and neurofeedback, not merely as therapeutic interventions but as catalysts for a deeper engagement with the self. They reveal a truth at the heart of these practices: that within the intricate systems of the body and the complex circuitry of the brain lies the potential for healing and growth, awaiting activation through awareness and intention. This potential, once unlocked, opens doors to realms of emotional and mental health that transcend conventional boundaries, offering hope and healing to those who tread its paths.

The journey through biofeedback and neurofeedback is, at its essence, a dialogue between technology and the self, a partnership where each session builds upon the last, mapping a route to emotional regulation and cognitive enhancement. It is a process marked by patience, for the changes it fosters, though profound, are often gradual, requiring persistence and dedication. Yet, for those who navigate this path, the rewards are manifold, manifesting in the ability to live with greater calm, focus, and resilience.

In this context, biofeedback and neurofeedback stand not merely as methods or techniques but as invitations to a deeper understanding of the self, to a place where control over one's internal landscape is not an abstract ideal but a lived reality. They offer a testament to the human capacity for adaptation and growth, highlighting a future where the boundaries of mental health and emotional well-being are continually expanded through the integration of technology and human endeavor.

7.4 THE HEALING POWER OF BREATHWORK

In the vast expanse of health and wellness practices, breathwork occupies a unique position, bridging the realms of the tangible and the ethereal, the conscious and the subconscious. This discipline, rooted in ancient traditions yet enduring in its relevance, centers on the deliberate manipulation of breath patterns to elicit specific physiological and psychological responses. The spectrum of techniques under the breathwork umbrella spans from the rhythmic tranquility of pranayama, a cornerstone of yoga, to the dynamic intensities of Holotropic and Rebirthing breathwork, methodologies developed in the latter half of the 20th century that emphasize rapid, deep breathing to promote emotional release and self-discovery.

At its core, breathwork serves as a conduit for enhancing oxygenation, a process fundamental to the vitality of every cell within the human body. By expanding lung capacity and optimizing the efficiency of the respiratory system, these practices ensure that greater volumes of oxygen reach the bloodstream, nourishing tissues and organs and facilitating the removal of carbon dioxide and other metabolic waste products. This enhanced oxygenation fosters not only physical rejuvenation but also mental clarity, as the brain, a voracious consumer of oxygen, operates with heightened efficiency in well-oxygenated environments.

The implications of breathwork for stress reduction and autonomic nervous system regulation are profound. Through techniques that deepen and slow the breath, practitioners can activate the parasympathetic nervous system, the body's innate mechanism for rest and repair. This shift away from the stress-induced activation of the sympathetic nervous system has tangible benefits, including reduced heart rate, lowered blood pressure, and a state of calm that permeates both mind and body. This balance between the sympathetic and parasympathetic branches, crucial for health and well-being, underscores the potential of breathwork as a powerful tool for stress management and emotional regulation.

For those embarking on the path of breathwork, adherence to safe practices is paramount. Beginners might find solace in guided sessions that introduce foundational techniques, such as diaphragmatic breathing or alternate nostril breathing, in a structured, supportive environment. These initial forays into breathwork should prioritize comfort and gradual progression, allowing individuals to acclimate to the sensations and experiences that accompany intensive breathing practices. As proficiency grows, so too can the complexity and intensity of the techniques, with advanced practices offering deeper insights into the psyche and enhanced physical resilience.

The connection between breathwork and longevity cannot be understated, with empirical evidence underscoring its potential to mitigate factors contributing to premature aging. Studies have illuminated the capacity of regular breathwork practice to reduce markers of oxidative stress and inflammation, conditions implicated in the pathogenesis of a myriad of chronic diseases. Furthermore, the role of breathwork in bolstering immune function through mechanisms is still the subject of ongoing research, which suggests an additional avenue by which these practices contribute to a longer, healthier life.

In the final analysis, breathwork stands as a testament to the power of the breath, a force so intrinsic to life yet so often overlooked in its potential for healing and transformation. This exploration of breathwork, from its diverse techniques and origins to its profound benefits for physical and mental health, invites a reevaluation of the breath as a tool for personal and physiological enhancement. It underscores the simplicity and accessibility of breathwork as a modality for wellness, one that requires no equipment, no special setting, but merely the willingness to turn inward and harness the life-giving force that flows through each inhalation and exhalation.

As we close this discussion, the essence of breathwork as a pathway to health, balance, and longevity crystallizes, offering a beacon for those seeking to navigate the complexities of modern life with grace and vitality. It invites a deeper engagement with the self through the most basic yet profound act of living: breathing. In this recognition lies the foundation for a practice that transcends mere technique, becoming a way of life, a rhythm that echoes the pulse of existence itself. Moving forward, the themes of connection, balance, and renewal that permeate this exploration of breathwork pave the way for a broader examination of wellness, one that integrates the physical, mental, and spiritual dimensions of health in pursuit of a life lived to its fullest potential.

DIGITAL HARMONY: RECLAIMING PRESENCE IN THE AGE OF DISTRACTION

In an era where the digital landscape continuously expands, enveloping our senses in a barrage of notifications, updates, and alerts, the act of disconnecting becomes an act of rebellion. A rebellion not against technology itself but against the pervasive intrusion of digital demands into the sanctuaries of our personal lives. This chapter delves into the essence of digital detoxing, a deliberate withdrawal from the digital web, aiming to restore balance and foster a more mindful interaction with our devices. It's an acknowledgment that while technology serves as a bridge to the world's knowledge and social connectivity, it also demands a toll on our mental, emotional, and physical well-being.

8.1 DIGITAL DETOXING: BALANCING TECHNOLOGY IN YOUR LIFE

The Impact of Digital Overload

The relentless barrage of digital stimuli—endless emails, the siren call of social media notifications, the beckoning of binge-worthy streaming services—exacts a subtle yet profound toll on our health. This constant connectivity, often heralded as a hallmark of modern efficiency, paradoxically engenders a state of perpetual distraction, diminishing our capacity for deep focus and undermining our mental tranquility. The symptoms of digital overload manifest not only in frayed nerves and diminished attention spans but in the erosion of our ability to engage in the reflective, uninterrupted thought critical for creativity and problem-solving.

Principles of a Digital Detox

A digital detox, contrary to misconceptions, is not an outright renunciation of technology but a strategic retreat, allowing us to reassess and recalibrate our relationship with digital devices. It's predicated on the understanding that moderation, rather than abstinence, fosters a sustainable harmony between our online and offline lives. The essence of this approach lies in mindful usage—recognizing when technology serves us and when it ensnares us in a web of compulsive engagement.

Benefits of Periodic Digital Breaks

Periodic disengagement from the digital realm unveils a multitude of benefits akin to the rejuvenation one feels after a nature retreat. Freed from the constant pull of notifications, our minds reclaim the silence necessary for introspection and creativity. Relationships, too, flourish under the undivided attention undiluted by the presence of screens, fostering deeper connections. Moreover, the practice of digital breaks, especially before bedtime, can significantly enhance sleep quality, liberating us from the blue light that disrupts our circadian rhythms and the mental stimulation that wards off sleep.

Implementing Digital Boundaries

Creating a healthier relationship with technology starts with setting clear, achievable boundaries. One might designate tech-free zones within the home, sanctuaries where devices are unwelcome, or tech-free hours, periods dedicated to unwinding and engaging in non-digital activities. For instance, meal times can transform into opportunities for undistracted conversations, and bedrooms can revert to havens of rest, free from the glow and buzz of smartphones. Implementing these boundaries requires not just individual resolve but collective respect, necessitating open dialogue with family members to foster a shared commitment to these digital-free oases.

Visual Element: Daily Digital Detox Checklist

A visual checklist serves as a daily reminder of small, actionable steps toward minimizing digital intrusion. This checklist might include tasks such as "Turn off non-essential notifications," "Commit to no screens 1 hour before bedtime," and "Engage in at least one tech-free leisure activity." By ticking off these tasks throughout the day, individuals can visually track their progress, reinforcing the detox habits and gradually weaving them into the fabric of daily life.

In navigating the currents of the digital age, the concept of detoxing transcends the act of disconnection, evolving into a practice of mindful reconnection with the world around us. It reminds us that in the cacophony of digital noise, the most profound connections often arise in silence, in the moments we choose to look up from our screens and engage with life unfiltered. Through the principles and practices of digital detoxing, we learn not just to coexist with technology but to command it, ensuring that our digital interactions augment rather than diminish the quality of our lives.

8.2 THE IMPACT OF ENVIRONMENTAL TOXINS ON HEALTH

In the tapestry of wellness and longevity, the silent threads of environmental toxins weave a complex pattern, often overlooked yet insidiously pervasive. These toxins, invisible assailants, permeate the air we breathe, the water we drink, and the very walls that shelter us, contributing to a spectrum of health dilemmas that range from subtle to severe. Identifying the sources of these environmental pollutants becomes a crucial first step in mitigating their impact on our health. Common culprits include volatile organic compounds (VOCs) emanating from paints, furniture, and building materials; pesticides lingering on non-organic produce; heavy metals like lead and mercury seeping into water supplies; and plasticizers such as bisphenol A (BPA) leaching from containers into our food and beverages. Each of these substances carries the potential for harm, disrupting bodily functions and contributing to chronic conditions.

Strategies for reducing exposure to harmful substances pivot around awareness and proactive measures. Initiatives such as opting for low-VOC or VOC-free paints and sustainable building materials can significantly lower the burden of airborne toxins within living spaces. Similarly, selecting organic produce and filtering drinking water become acts of self-preservation, minimizing the ingestion of pesticides and heavy metals. In the realm of consumer goods, favoring products free from BPA and phthalates, particularly in items that come into direct contact with food, further reduces the toxic load our bodies must contend with. These steps, though simple in concept, require a shift towards conscious consumption, a commitment to prioritizing health in every purchase, and lifestyle choice.

Detoxifying your living space emerges as an extension of this commitment, transforming the home into a sanctuary from environmental pollutants. Beyond the selection of materials and products that minimize toxin exposure, regular practices such as thorough ventilation to dispel accumulated indoor air pollutants and the incorporation of indoor plants that act as natural air purifiers contribute to a healthier living environment. The use of high-efficiency particulate air (HEPA) filters in vacuum cleaners and air purification systems offers another layer of defense, trapping airborne particles, including allergens, mold spores, and particulate matter, thereby enhancing the quality of the air that circulates within our homes.

The role of diet and lifestyle in detoxification represents a critical pillar in the edifice of wellness, offering the body's natural cleansing systems the support they need to function optimally. Incorporating foods rich in antioxidants, fibers, and essential nutrients bolsters the liver and kidneys, organs at the forefront of detoxification efforts, enhancing their ability to process and eliminate toxins. Cruciferous vegetables such as broccoli and Brussels sprouts, rich in compounds that support liver enzymes, along with fruits high in antioxidants and fibers, such as berries and apples, play starring roles in the detoxification diet. Hydration, too, stands paramount, facilitating the elimination of waste products through urine and sweat. Engaging in regular physical activity further supports detoxification processes, improving circulation and encouraging the elimination of toxins through sweat.

Moreover, adopting lifestyle habits that reduce the production of endogenous toxins—those generated within the body—complements external detoxification efforts. Stress management techniques such as meditation and yoga not only counteract the negative effects of stress hormones but also mitigate the internal biochemical disturbances they cause. Adequate sleep, by supporting the restorative functions of the glymphatic system, a waste clearance system in the brain, plays an indispensable role in preventing the accumulation of neurotoxic waste products.

In navigating the landscape of environmental toxins, our actions, informed by awareness and guided by intention, become our most potent tools. The choices we make, from the foods we consume to the materials we surround ourselves with, craft a personal environment that either burdens or supports our body's intrinsic capacity for detoxification. Through the vigilant selection of products, conscious dietary habits, and a lifestyle attuned to wellness, we construct a bulwark against the insidious impact of environmental toxins, safeguarding our health and enhancing our journey toward longevity. In this endeavor, the alliance between knowledge and action emerges not merely as a strategy but as a fundamental principle, propelling us toward a life marked not by the passive accumulation of toxins but by the active cultivation of vitality.

8.3 STRATEGIES FOR MANAGING INFORMATION OVERLOAD

In the labyrinth of the modern world, where information proliferates with relentless velocity, the human mind finds itself at the nexus of endless streams of data, each vying for attention. While a testament to humanity's insatiable quest for knowledge, this deluge paradoxically engenders a state of cognitive disarray, diminishing our capacity to discern, digest, and derive meaning from the vastness of available content. The phenomenon, known as information overload, exacts a toll on psychological well-being, fostering a milieu where stress and distraction undermine the serenity and focus essential for meaningful engagement with life.

At the heart of mitigating this cognitive and emotional quagmire lies the art of filtering, a deliberate process of curating the influx of information to align with personal relevance and capacity. Tools and applications designed with sophisticated algorithms offer gateways to manage the flow, allowing individuals to tailor their digital environments to reflect priorities and interests. Email filters, social media curation tools, and news aggregators become custodians of our attention, sifting through the chaff to present the kernels of information that resonate with our quests and curiosities. Yet, beyond the utility of technological aids, the practice of filtering necessitates an introspective clarity, a conscious recognition of the themes and narratives that truly enrich our lives.

Equally pivotal to navigating the torrents of information is the cultivation of mindful consumption, an approach that transcends passive reception to foster an active, discerning engagement with content. This mindfulness, rooted in the ancient wisdom of presence, invites a pause, a moment of reflection before the act of consumption, prompting questions of value and utility. It encourages a shift from the quantitative accumulation of facts to a qualitative immersion in knowledge, where depth supersedes breadth, and understanding eclipses mere awareness. In this space, media consumption transforms into a deliberate act imbued with intention and purpose, fostering a relationship with information that nourishes rather than depletes.

The construction of an information management plan emerges as a strategic blueprint to reclaim autonomy over our cognitive landscapes. This plan, tailored to individual rhythms and life demands, outlines structured intervals for engagement with digital media, interspersed with sanctuaries of silence and disconnection. It advocates for the allocation of specific times for email correspondence, social media interaction, and news consumption, framing these activities within boundaries that preserve the sanctity of concentration and the richness of the unmediated experience. Moreover, the plan emphasizes the ritual of daily reviews, moments set aside to reflect on the information absorbed, assimilating insights and weaving them into the fabric of our understanding and actions. Through these practices, the information management plan serves not as a rigid set of rules but as a fluid framework, adaptable to the evolving dynamics of our lives and the shifting landscapes of the digital domain.

In the endeavor to mitigate information overload, the strategies delineated herein converge on a singular imperative: the restoration of agency in an age of ubiquity. They summon a recalibration of our interactions with the digital world, invoking a paradigm where serenity and depth of thought reclaim their rightful place at the forefront of our existence. By meticulously curating the information we allow into our mental space, the mindful engagement with the media we consume, and the strategic planning of our digital interactions, we navigate the complexities of the information age. In this navigation, we discover the means to alleviate the burden of overload and the pathways to a richer, more meaningful exchange with the world of knowledge that surrounds us.

8.4 SLEEP HYGIENE FOR THE 21ST CENTURY

In this epoch where the boundaries between day and night blur under the glare of perpetual connectivity, the sanctity of sleep has been besieged by an armada of modern lifestyle disruptors. From the blue light emissions of our cherished devices to the cacophony of a 24/7 lifestyle, each element insidiously encroaches upon the realm of rest, fragmenting the architecture of sleep that our ancestors once took for granted. This section navigates through the intricate dance of reclaiming the night, piecing together the fragmented shards of restorative slumber in an age that seldom sleeps.

The landscape of contemporary sleep challenges is vast, marked by the omnipresence of screens that emit a spectrum of light mimicking the midday sun, tricking our brains into a state of perpetual alertness. Caffeine, a revered elixir of wakefulness, now flows abundantly beyond the morning hours, extending its reach into the night, further muddying the waters of our circadian rhythms. The relentless pace of modern life itself, with its late-night work emails and the siren call of binge-watching, compounds the siege, rendering the pursuit of sleep a nightly battle against the very fabric of contemporary existence.

Against this backdrop, the principles of good sleep hygiene emerge as beacons of hope, guiding principles that light the way back to the restorative embrace of sleep. These principles advocate for a sanctification of the sleep environment—transforming bedrooms into minimalist havens of tranquility, free from the electronic devices that fracture our rest. They speak to the rhythm of sleep rituals, gentle preludes to slumber involving soothing activities that signal the brain to wind down, be it through the pages of a book or the melody of soft music. Temperature, too, plays a critical role in this ballet of sleep, with the ideal conditions mirroring the cool embrace of the night air, a subtle cue to the body that the time for rest has arrived.

The thread that weaves through the narrative of sleep and longevity is one of profound interconnection, a dialogue between rest and vitality that science has only begun to decipher fully. Studies proliferate, drawing lines of correlation between the quality and quantity of sleep and the vast expanse of health outcomes. Research delineates how deep, restorative sleep acts as a cornerstone of immune function, a time when the body repairs and rejuvenates at a cellular level. It highlights sleep's role as a custodian of cognitive health, safeguarding memory and executive function against the erosion of time. In this light, sleep transcends its traditional domain, heralded not merely as a period of inactivity but as an active participant in the body's pursuit of longevity.

Tailoring sleep strategies to the individual tapestry of needs and challenges becomes an art form in its own right, a personalized approach to reclaiming the night. For those ensnared by the tendrils of insomnia, strategies might involve cognitive-behavioral therapy for insomnia (CBT-I), a structured program that addresses the thoughts and behaviors that hinder sleep. For others, adjusting sleep schedules to align with natural circadian rhythms offers a path to synchronization with the internal clock, enhancing both sleep quality and daytime vitality. The intervention of technology, para-doxically, can also serve sleep, with apps designed to foster relax-ation through guided meditations or the generation of white noise, crafting an auditory cocoon from which sleep can emerge unen-cumbered.

In navigating the nuanced landscape of sleep in the digital age, the principles outlined herein converge on a singular truth: that in the stillness of the night lies the wellspring of vitality that nourishes the day. Through the sanctification of our sleep environments, the culti-vation of pre-sleep rituals, the embrace of science-backed strategies for sleep enhancement, and the personalization of our approach to rest, we forge a path back to the restorative embrace of sleep. This journey, marked by an understanding of sleep's pivotal role in health and longevity, invites a rekindling of our relationship with the night, a reclamation of our right to rest, and a renewal of our commitment to the holistic pursuit of well-being.

As we close this exploration of sleep hygiene in the digital era, it becomes evident that the journey toward optimal health is multifaceted, requiring attention not only to the foods we eat and the air we breathe but also to the sacred realm of sleep. In understanding and addressing the challenges that modern life poses to our rest and in adopting strategies to enhance the quality of our sleep, we lay the foundation for a life of vitality and longevity. This acknowledgment of sleep's central role in our well-being seamlessly leads us into the broader exploration of lifestyle habits that support health and longevity, underscoring the interconnectedness of all aspects of our lives in the pursuit of wellness.

NURTURING THE SELF: A BLUEPRINT FOR PERSONALIZED WELLNESS

In an age where the mirage of quick fixes and universal solutions often clouds the path to true wellness, the act of turning inward to assess one's unique health aspirations marks the beginning of a genuine transformation. This self-assessment, far from a mere inventory of physical capabilities or limitations, invites a deep dive into the reservoirs of one's desires, fears, and hopes, setting the stage for a wellness strategy that resonates with the individual's core. It is here, in the quiet reflection on personal health priorities, that the foundation for a lasting journey towards optimal well-being is laid, brick by brick, with intention and insight.

9.1 ASSESSING YOUR HEALTH AND WELLNESS GOALS

Identifying Personal Health Priorities

The process of reflection on one's health status and aspirations is akin to an artist standing before a blank canvas, contemplating the masterpiece to emerge. This moment, brimming with potential, requires an honest evaluation of where one stands and where one wishes to go. A useful exercise involves listing current health concerns, be it managing stress, improving sleep quality, or enhancing physical fitness, alongside aspirations that range from running a marathon to cultivating a practice of daily mindfulness. This list, a mosaic of needs and dreams, serves as a compass, guiding the subsequent steps on this path.

Setting SMART Goals for Wellness

The art of goal-setting, when approached with the SMART framework, transforms nebulous aspirations into tangible targets. Specific, Measurable, Achievable, Relevant, and Time-bound goals carve a clear pathway through the often overwhelming terrain of wellness improvement. For instance, instead of a vague intention to "get fit," a SMART goal articulates a precise aim: "To increase my jogging distance to 5 kilometers within the next three months by adding half a kilometer every week." This clarity not only sharpens focus but also elevates motivation, making the abstract concrete.

Holistic Approach to Wellness Goals

In the crafting of wellness goals, the inclusion of mental, emotional, and spiritual objectives alongside physical ones acknowledges the intricate tapestry of human health. This holistic perspective recognizes that true well-being is not merely the absence of illness but a harmonious balance of the physical with the psychological and spiritual dimensions. A goal might, therefore, encompass practices that nurture the mind and spirit, such as dedicating fifteen minutes each morning to journaling or meditation, enriching the journey with depth and breadth.

Adjusting Goals Over Time

Flexibility in pursuing wellness allows for the natural ebb and flow of life's circumstances. Goals set at the outset are not cast in stone but are signposts that can be shifted as needed. This adaptability ensures that the wellness strategy remains relevant and responsive to the individual's evolving needs, aspirations, and challenges. Regular check-ins, perhaps monthly or quarterly, serve as opportunities to reassess and recalibrate goals, ensuring they remain aligned with one's current reality and vision for the future.

Visual Element: Wellness Goal-Setting Template

A structured template for setting and tracking wellness goals, presented as an interactive PDF, offers a practical tool for individuals to articulate their aspirations in the SMART format. This template, designed for ease of use, includes sections detailing specific goals, actions to achieve them, potential obstacles, and strategies for overcoming these hurdles. By filling out this template, individuals can visualize their path to wellness, monitor progress, and make necessary adjustments, turning abstract aspirations into achievable plans.

In this approach to assessing health and wellness goals, the emphasis on personalization, clarity, and flexibility resonates with the understanding that each individual's path to optimal health is unique. The process of setting SMART goals, grounded in a holistic perspective and adaptable over time, equips individuals with a clear, actionable blueprint for their wellness journey. It is through this meticulous planning and reflection that the seeds of transformation are sown and nurtured by the individual's commitment to their health and well-being.

9.2 INTEGRATING BIOHACKS INTO YOUR DAILY ROUTINE

In optimizing one's health through the lens of modern science and age-old wisdom, the concept of biohacking emerges as a beacon for those seeking to fine-tune their physiological and psychological well-being. This endeavor requires not merely the adoption of novel practices but a discerning approach that tailors these interventions to meet the nuanced demands of individual lifestyles and health aspirations. Personalizing biohacks, therefore, becomes not just a strategy but a necessity, ensuring that each modification to one's routine resonates with their unique health blueprint and life's rhythm.

Choosing biohacks that align with specific health goals and lifestyle constraints necessitates an analytical yet intuitive process akin to a sculptor selecting tools that best shape the raw material at hand. For individuals grappling with stress-induced maladies, biohacks that recalibrate the body's stress response, such as controlled breathing techniques or cold exposure, offer a starting point. Conversely, those navigating the complexities of disrupted sleep patterns might find solace in red-light therapy or the strategic use of blue-light blockers. This bespoke approach underscores the importance of understanding the underlying mechanics of each biohack, allowing individuals to match these interventions with their health objectives and daily schedules.

For novices in the biohacking sphere, the initiation into this practice benefits from simplicity, focusing on biohacks that demand minimal investment yet yield significant returns. The act of hydrating immediately upon waking, leveraging the body's overnight fasting state to reset and rehydrate, serves as a foundational yet powerful biohack. Similarly, integrating a short midday sunlight exposure nurtures circadian rhythms, bolstering sleep quality and mood with minimal effort. These simple interventions, easily woven into the fabric of daily life, lay the groundwork for a more nuanced exploration of biohacking techniques, setting the stage for the gradual incorporation of more advanced practices.

As individuals gain fluency in these initial biohacks, the landscape expands, inviting the integration of more sophisticated techniques for those ready to amplify their wellness regimen. The exploration of fasting protocols, from intermittent fasting to more extended fasts, offers a deeper dive into metabolic flexibility and autophagy, processes linked with longevity and healthspan. The utilization of nootropics, substances that enhance cognitive function, requires a meticulous approach, balancing efficacy with safety, to ensure these cognitive enhancers complement rather than compromise one's health objectives. This progression from foundational to advanced biohacks mirrors the journey of mastery in any domain, where complexity builds upon a bedrock of fundamental principles.

A harmonious approach emerges as paramount when navigating the confluence of modern biohacking techniques and traditional health practices. This balance honors the innovation that biohacking brings to the wellness domain while acknowledging the timeless efficacy of conventional health modalities. For instance, the modern practice of using technology to track sleep patterns can be complemented by the traditional wisdom of herbal teas known for their soothing properties. Similarly, the advanced biohack of using specific dietary supplements to enhance mitochondrial function finds its counterpart in the practice of consuming nutrient-dense whole foods—a principle espoused by dietary traditions across cultures. This synthesis of cutting-edge and time-honored practices broadens the spectrum of wellness strategies at one's disposal and fosters a holistic view of health, where innovation and tradition merge to support the body and mind.

In the pursuit of personalizing biohacks, the guiding principle remains a steadfast commitment to self-awareness and adaptability, recognizing that the efficacy of any health intervention is ultimately measured by its resonance with the individual's unique physiological and psychological landscape. This approach, grounded in discernment and flexibility, ensures that biohacking transcends the realm of mere experimentation to become a tailored strategy for enhancing life quality. Herein lies the art of integrating biohacks into daily routines, a dynamic process that marries science with intuition, modernity with tradition, and innovation with wisdom in the continual quest for optimal well-being.

9.3 SETTING REALISTIC, ACHIEVABLE HEALTH MILESTONES

In pursuing a life augmented by vitality and devoid of ailment, the crafting of milestones serves as beacons that guide the way through the fog of ambition toward the shores of accomplishment. The meticulous division of overarching aspirations into bite-sized, attainable objectives acts as a scaffold upon which the edifice of comprehensive well-being is constructed. This methodical deconstruction of grand ambitions into smaller, actionable segments ensures that the path to wellness remains clear, navigable, and imbued with a sense of progress at every turn.

The recognition and celebration of incremental achievements imbue the wellness odyssey with a sense of momentum, transforming the journey from a daunting expedition into a series of rewarding, achievable quests. Each minor victory, be it the consistent hydration over the course of a week, the successful integration of a five-minute meditation practice into the morning routine, or the addition of a new vegetable into the diet, merits acknowledgment. This act of celebration, far from a mere pat on the back, serves as a potent motivator, reinforcing the positive behaviors that contribute to the larger vision of health and well-being. It is in these moments of reflection and jubilation that the belief in one's ability to effect change is fortified, propelling the individual forward with renewed vigor and conviction.

The path to transformation, however, is seldom linear, marked as it is by the inevitable presence of hurdles and setbacks. The recalibration of expectations to accommodate the realities of human nature and the unpredictability of life is not an admission of defeat but a strategic pivot toward sustainability. Acceptance of the fact that change is incremental and that setbacks are not regressions but part of the learning and growth process fosters resilience. It tempers the impatience for immediate results with the wisdom to appreciate the journey itself, understanding that cultivating health is not a race but a lifelong endeavor that demands patience, persistence, and a compassionate understanding of self.

Encountering obstacles along the wellness path is an inevitability that tests resolve, patience, and adaptability. The strategies employed to navigate these challenges determine not only the immediate outcome but the long-term sustainability of health improvements. A foundational strategy lies in the anticipatory identification of potential barriers, be they environmental temptations, social pressures, or internal conflicts, and the pre-emptive crafting of countermeasures. This proactive approach ensures that when faced with hurdles, the individual is not caught unawares but is equipped with a repertoire of responses that mitigate the impact of these challenges.

A critical component of overcoming setbacks is cultivating a support system, a collective of like-minded individuals, mentors, and confidants who offer encouragement, advice, and accountability. This network acts as a safety net, providing emotional and motivational support during moments of doubt and reinforcing the commitment to wellness goals. Furthermore, the adoption of a mindset that views obstacles not as insurmountable barriers but as opportunities for learning and growth transforms the approach to setbacks. It shifts the narrative from one of failure to one of exploration, where each challenge is dissected to extract valuable insights that inform future strategies, refining the approach to health and wellness with each iteration.

In this intricate dance of setting milestones, celebrating achievements, recalibrating expectations, and surmounting setbacks, the journey toward optimal health evolves into a tapestry rich with experience, learning, and personal growth. Segmenting goals into manageable steps ensures that the path remains accessible and achievable, imbued with a sense of progress and accomplishment that fuels motivation. The celebration of small wins nourishes the spirit, enhancing the resilience needed to face and learn from the inevitable challenges that arise. Through this nuanced approach to wellness, marked by strategic planning, adaptability, and a supportive community, the pursuit of health transcends the realm of physicality to become a journey of self-discovery, empowerment, and transformation.

9.4 TRACKING PROGRESS: TOOLS AND TECHNOLOGIES

In the nuanced tapestry of personal wellness, monitoring progress transcends mere vanity, serving as a cornerstone for informed decision-making and strategic adjustments. This meticulous observation, facilitated by the advent of sophisticated apps, wearable devices, and online platforms, provides a multidimensional view of health metrics, painting a vivid portrait of where one stands on the spectrum of wellness. These digital companions, each equipped with the ability to track everything from caloric intake and sleep patterns to heart rate variability and exercise frequency, serve as silent witnesses to our daily habits, offering insights that guide the fine-tuning of personal health strategies.

Beyond the realm of digital trackers lies the venerable practice of journaling, a method steeped in introspection and self-discovery. This practice, far removed from the quantifiable metrics of apps and wearables, invites a deeper dive into the qualitative aspects of well-being. By penning down thoughts, emotions, and experiences, individuals engage in a dialogue with themselves, uncovering patterns and insights that might elude even the most advanced technological trackers. This reflective process, while subjective, complements the objective data collected by digital tools, providing a holistic view of progress that encompasses the physical, mental, and emotional dimensions of health.

Navigating the intersection of quantitative and qualitative measures of success requires a delicate balance, acknowledging that numbers can illuminate trends but not the richness of the human experience. While a wearable device might report an improvement in sleep quality, it is the individual's subjective feeling of restfulness upon waking that completes the picture. Similarly, a journal entry describing a sense of accomplishment after a month of consistent meditation adds depth to the data, capturing the emotional and psychological benefits that numbers might not fully convey. This symbiosis between data-driven metrics and subjective assessments forms the bedrock of a comprehensive wellness monitoring strategy, ensuring that both the tangible and intangible aspects of health are accounted for.

Amidst the embrace of technology as an ally in wellness monitoring, considerations surrounding privacy and data security emerge as paramount. The intimate nature of health-related data demands a cautious approach to sharing and storing this information. Opting for apps and platforms that prioritize user privacy, employing robust encryption methods, and being judicious about the permissions granted to these applications can mitigate the risk of unauthorized access to personal health information. Moreover, regularly reviewing and managing privacy settings, coupled with a discerning eye for the terms of service of digital health tools, ensures that one's health data remains a closely guarded asset, accessible only to those with explicit permission.

As this exploration of monitoring tools and strategies draws to a close, the tapestry of wellness tracking reveals itself not as a static picture but as a dynamic mosaic, continuously shaped by the interplay of technology, introspection, and personal growth. The judicious use of apps and wearable devices offers a window into the quantifiable aspects of health, while journaling and self-reflection add color and texture to this picture, capturing the nuanced shades of well-being. Balancing these quantitative and qualitative measures ensures a rich, multifaceted understanding of progress, one that honors the complexity of the human condition. Privacy and data security considerations serve as the frame for this mosaic, delineating the boundaries within which this personal exploration unfolds, safeguarding the sanctity of our health data as we navigate the path to optimal well-being.

In the grand scheme, the meticulous tracking of wellness progress, facilitated by an array of tools and tempered by introspection, embodies a commitment to self-awareness and continuous improvement. It is a testament to the belief that in the meticulous observation of our habits, responses, and experiences lies the key to unlocking a deeper understanding of ourselves, guiding us toward a state of health that resonates with our deepest aspirations. As we transition from the detailed examination of tracking methodologies, the narrative shifts towards the broader landscape of community and support in wellness, reminding us that while the journey to health is deeply personal, it is also inextricably linked to the world around us, enriched by the connections we forge and the shared pursuit of a life lived to its fullest potential.

CULTIVATING COLLECTIVE WELLNESS: A SYMPHONY OF SUPPORT

In the orchestration of wellness, the solo pursuit of health often finds its melody enriched by the harmonious contributions of a community. This collective symphony, where the support and camaraderie of others amplify each individual's efforts, transforms the solitary act of self-improvement into a shared endeavor, resonating with the power of unity. Within this ensemble, the role of community not only acts as a catalyst for personal growth but also as a bastion of motivation and accountability, guiding each member towards their highest aspirations of health and well-being.

10.1 BUILDING A SUPPORTIVE WELLNESS COMMUNITY

Finding Like-minded Individuals

The quest to connect with those who share similar health and wellness goals begins in the most unassuming of places. Consider the local gym, a place where personal goals drive each member, yet a collective energy permeates the space, creating an environment ripe for connection. These spaces, along with virtual forums dedicated to wellness topics, serve as fertile ground for the seeds of community to take root. Engaging in discussions about the best post-workout recovery practices or strategies for maintaining a balanced diet fosters a sense of camaraderie and shared purpose. The act of reaching out, both physically in community events and digitally through social media groups focused on wellness, cultivates a network of peers who offer not just advice but encouragement and understanding.

The Power of Group Accountability

There's undeniable strength in numbers. This principle holds true in wellness, where the journey's challenges often require a reservoir of motivation and support. Accountability groups, whether formal or informal, act as a compass, keeping each member oriented toward their goals. A simple weekly check-in, sharing successes and setbacks, becomes a ritual of reflection and recalibration. This shared accountability, much like a pact among climbers tethered together, ensures that no one strays too far from the path without the supportive pull of the group guiding them back.

Creating or Joining Wellness-focused Groups

The inception of a wellness group, or the decision to join one, marks a pivotal step in the communal wellness journey. Starting a group might begin with a call to action within a yoga class, inviting participants to form a weekly meditation circle, extending the sense of peace from the mat to the complexities of daily life. For those seeking established groups, local community centers often host a variety of wellness activities, from running clubs to healthy cooking workshops, providing ready-made communities eager to welcome new members. The key lies in aligning the group's focus with one's personal wellness goals, ensuring a symbiotic relationship that nurtures growth and fosters a sense of belonging.

Leveraging Community Resources

The wealth of knowledge and opportunities within a community often goes untapped, overlooked amidst the bustle of daily routines. Yet, within this reservoir lies a multitude of resources poised to support wellness goals. Libraries, for example, not only offer literature on nutrition and fitness but also host seminars and talks by wellness experts. Local parks, with their open spaces and trails, invite physical activity amidst nature's calming presence. Even community colleges serve as hubs of learning, offering courses on stress management, holistic health, and more. The act of seeking out and utilizing these resources not only enriches one's wellness journey but also strengthens the connection to the community, fostering a shared commitment to health and well-being.

The endeavor to weave the fabric of a supportive wellness community, rich with the threads of shared aspirations, accountability, and resources, underscores the profound impact of collective efforts on individual health journeys. In this communal symphony, each member's contribution, whether a note of encouragement or a melody of shared experiences, harmonizes into a chorus that uplifts and inspires, driving the collective towards a crescendo of wellness and vitality.

10.2 THE BENEFITS OF GROUP EXERCISE AND SOCIAL ACTIVITIES

Group fitness transcends the boundaries of mere physical exertion, weaving into its fabric an intricate network of psychological reinforcements and communal bonds that elevate the practice into a holistic experience. Within this collective endeavor, participants discover the fortification of their physical capabilities and the cultivation of a shared resilience, a mutual energy that propels each member forward, surmounting the inevitable plateaus and valleys of the fitness landscape. This communal resilience, born from synchronized effort and shared triumphs, fosters a sense of belonging and achievement, enhancing the individual's commitment to sustained physical activity and its benefits.

Variety marks the essence of group exercise offerings, catering to a spectrum of interests and capabilities, from the serene flow of yoga sessions that invite introspection and flexibility to the dynamic rhythms of dance classes that celebrate movement and expression. The resurgence of outdoor boot camps, marrying the rigor of structured exercise with the spontaneity of nature's backdrop, offers an alternative for those seeking the vitality of fresh air alongside the camaraderie of like-minded enthusiasts. For individuals drawn to the challenges of endurance and strength, cycling clubs and running groups provide a platform for the collective pursuit of personal bests, where encouragement and shared experience dilute the strain of exertion. This diversity ensures that within group exercise, each individual finds a niche, a space where personal health aspirations align with activities that resonate, ensuring engagement and persistence.

At the core of shared wellness activities lies the potential for forging deep, meaningful connections, a phenomenon that transcends the confines of traditional social interactions. As individuals sweat, laugh, and strive together, barriers dissolve, unveiling the raw, authentic selves hidden beneath social facades. This vulnerability becomes the soil from which strong, supportive relationships sprout, nurtured by mutual respect and the shared journey toward better health. These connections, forged in the crucible of collective struggle and triumph, extend beyond the parameters of the exercise session, spilling into the realm of daily life, where they continue to flourish, providing a network of support and encouragement.

Community-led wellness initiatives exemplify the power of collective action in transforming the health landscape of neighborhoods and cities. These programs, often sprouting from the grassroots level, harness the collective will of residents to institute change, from the establishment of community gardens that provide access to fresh, nutritious produce to the organization of neighborhood 'walkabouts' that promote physical activity while fostering social connectivity. Urban areas, previously marked by the anonymity of high-density living, witness the emergence of running clubs that reclaim the streets for the feet of residents, transforming thoroughfares into trails of camaraderie. Similarly, workplaces, recognizing the integral role of physical health in overall employee well-being and productivity, have begun to champion corporate wellness programs that encourage group exercise, from on-site fitness classes to sponsored participation in local fitness events. These initiatives amplify the benefits of physical activity through the power of community and reframe the narrative of health from an individual pursuit to a collective endeavor, where each person's wellness journey contributes to a larger tapestry of communal health.

The narrative unfolds in exploring the benefits of group exercise and social activities, revealing the multidimensional impact of communal physical endeavors. Here, the pursuit of fitness becomes a shared voyage, where the physical benefits of exercise meld with the psychological uplift of belonging and the emotional richness of new friendships. This collective experience, marked by diversity, connectivity, and community engagement, redefines the concept of wellness, presenting it not as a solitary quest but as a communal celebration of health, vitality, and human connection.

10.3 VOLUNTEERING: GIVING BACK FOR YOUR HEALTH

In the intricate dance of life, where individual aspirations often lead the choreography, the act of volunteering emerges as a profound counterpoint, a movement that extends the self beyond the confines of personal gain into the realm of altruistic giving. This pivot, seemingly outward, harbors a paradox at its core: in the giving of oneself, in the dedication of time and energy to causes beyond the individual, a wealth of health benefits, both mental and physical, is reaped. This section explores the multifaceted benefits of volunteering, not merely as an act of charity but as a pivotal component of holistic wellness.

The connection between altruistic behaviors and mental health has been well-documented, revealing a landscape where the selfless act of volunteering acts as a balm for the soul. Engaging in volunteer work provides a sense of purpose, a beacon that guides individuals through the fog of everyday routines and the malaise of existential questioning. When aligned with personal values and passions, this purpose ignites a sense of fulfillment that transcends the immediate gratification of individual achievements, offering a more profound, sustained sense of satisfaction. Furthermore, the social interactions inherent in most volunteer activities counter the isolation and loneliness plaguing contemporary society, offering a forum for meaningful connection and the development of empathetic relationships. These emotional and psychological benefits, in turn, contribute to a fortified sense of self-esteem as individuals witness the tangible impact of their efforts on the well-being of others and the community at large.

The pursuit of volunteer opportunities that resonate with one's wellness goals invites a deliberate selection process, a matching of personal aspirations with the needs of the community. For example, initiatives focused on environmental conservation allow individuals passionate about the outdoors to engage in activities that reinforce their connection to nature while contributing to the planet's health. Similarly, programs aimed at promoting physical activity among youth or older adults offer a platform for those dedicated to fitness to share their enthusiasm and expertise, fostering a culture of health that spans generations. This alignment ensures that the act of volunteering amplifies personal health objectives, creating a feedback loop where community service reinforces and extends individual wellness goals.

Physical fitness and mobility find unexpected allies in the realm of volunteering. Activities that demand physical exertion, from the restoration of community parks to the organization of charity runs, provide volunteers with opportunities to maintain and enhance their physical health. These endeavors, often communal and outdoors, offer a dynamic alternative to traditional exercise routines, embedding physical activity within the context of service and social engagement. The variability of tasks and the camaraderie among volunteers transform what might otherwise be a solitary fitness regimen into an enriching experience that feeds both body and soul.

At the heart of volunteering lies the reciprocal nature of giving and receiving, a dynamic interplay that blurs the lines between benefactor and beneficiary. This reciprocity extends beyond the immediate exchange of assistance for gratitude, encompassing a broader, more profound exchange that enriches personal and community health. Volunteers often report a sense of increased well-being, a reflection of the "helper's high," a state of euphoria, and heightened emotional well-being following selfless acts of kindness. This emotional uplift has tangible health implications, contributing to reduced stress levels, lower blood pressure, and a general sense of physical well-being. Communities, in turn, thrive under the care and dedication of volunteers, witnessing improvements in social cohesion, access to services, and the overall quality of life. This mutual enhancement, where personal health gains are mirrored by community well-being, underscores the inherent value of volunteering as an integral component of a holistic approach to health.

In the delicate balance of giving and receiving, volunteering emerges not as a peripheral activity but as a central pillar in the architecture of wellness. It offers a pathway to health that weaves together the threads of physical activity, mental engagement, and emotional fulfillment, creating a tapestry of well-being that extends far beyond the individual. Through volunteering, individuals step into a broader, interconnected world where their actions ripple outward, touching lives and transforming communities. In this expansive view, health becomes not just a personal attribute but a communal asset nurtured by the selfless contributions of individuals dedicated to serving others.

10.4 NURTURING RELATIONSHIPS FOR MENTAL AND EMOTIONAL HEALTH

In the labyrinth of human experience, the threads that bind us to one another in relationships are as crucial to our well-being as the air we breathe. This intricate web of connections, spanning the spectrum from fleeting acquaintances to the most intimate of bonds, forms the backdrop against which our lives unfold. Within this context, cultivating deep, meaningful relationships stands as a pillar of mental and emotional health, a beacon that lights the path toward a fulfilled and balanced life.

The Importance of Deep, Meaningful Connections

At the heart of human connection lies the profound truth that our interactions with others mirror the complexities of our inner selves.

Deep, meaningful relationships offer a mirror in which we see reflected not only our strengths but also our vulnerabilities. This reflective process, grounded in trust and mutual respect, fosters a sense of belonging and acceptance fundamental to our psychological well-being. Studies underscore the correlation between the quality of personal relationships and a wide range of health outcomes, suggesting that the depth of our connections significantly influences our stress levels, immune function, and longevity. The alchemy of deep relationships transforms the mundane into the extraordinary, imbuing our daily lives with a sense of purpose and joy.

Strategies for Strengthening Existing Relationships

Fortifying the bonds that tether us to friends, family, and partners requires a commitment to openness and ongoing communication. This endeavor begins with the willingness to listen actively, an art that involves more than the passive reception of words. It demands an immersion in the moment, an attunement to the subtleties of tone and body language that convey volumes beyond the spoken word. In this space of attentive listening, we offer our loved ones a gift of presence that validates their experiences and emotions, laying the groundwork for a deeper connection.

Equally important is the practice of expressing gratitude, a simple yet profound gesture that acknowledges the value and significance of others in our lives. This expression, whether through words, acts of kindness, or small tokens of appreciation, reinforces the bonds of affection and respect that underpin healthy relationships. Moreover, the shared pursuit of new experiences, from exploring new hobbies to traveling to unfamiliar places, injects vitality into relationships, creating shared memories that weave a richer, more textured narrative of companionship.

Expanding Social Circles Later in Life

The endeavor to broaden one's social circle in adulthood, often perceived as a daunting task, is vital for injecting fresh perspectives and energy into our lives. This expansion necessitates stepping beyond the comfort zones of established routines and embracing opportunities for interaction that life presents. Joining clubs or groups that align with personal interests offers a platform for meeting individuals who share similar passions, providing a natural context for developing new friendships. Moreover, volunteering serves as a conduit for connection, drawing together people of diverse backgrounds united by a common purpose.

The digital age, with its plethora of social interaction platforms, presents unprecedented opportunities for building connections. Online forums and social networks dedicated to specific interests or life stages offer a virtual meeting ground for individuals seeking to widen their social networks. However, transitioning from digital interaction to meaningful, real-world connections demands intentionality, a conscious effort to bridge the gap between online camaraderie and tangible relationships.

Managing Toxic Relationships

Navigating the murky waters of toxic relationships, characterized by patterns of manipulation, disrespect, or emotional neglect, requires courage and clarity. The first step in this process is the recognition of the signs of toxicity, an acknowledgment that certain relationships drain our emotional reserves rather than replenish them. This awareness paves the way for setting boundaries, a crucial mechanism for protecting our mental and emotional well-being. These boundaries, clearly communicated and consistently enforced, delineate the limits of acceptable behavior, signaling our refusal to be diminished by others' actions.

In instances where toxic relationships prove resistant to change despite clear communication and boundary-setting, disengagement becomes a necessary act of self-preservation. Though fraught with difficulty, this decision underscores a commitment to one's mental and emotional health, a declaration that we value ourselves too highly to remain in environments that undermine our well-being.

In the grand narrative of our lives, the relationships we nurture and the connections we forge form the bedrock of our mental and emotional health. This chapter has traversed the terrain of human connection, from cultivating deep, meaningful relationships to expanding social circles and managing toxic dynamics. Each step in this journey underscores the indelible link between our interactions with others and our overall well-being, highlighting the importance of intentionality in building and maintaining relationships that enrich our lives.

As we close this exploration, we are reminded that the quality of our relationships is a reflection of our engagement with the world around us. In nurturing these connections, we not only enhance our own lives but also contribute to the well-being of our communities, weaving a tapestry of support and understanding that spans the breadth of human experience. With this foundation, we turn our gaze to the horizon, ready to explore the next chapter in our journey toward a life of wellness and fulfillment.

SOOTHING THE SENSES: NATURE'S BALM FOR JOINT HEALTH

In the labyrinth of modern wellness, where every path promises relief and rejuvenation, the ancient wisdom of nature holds the key to unlocking a profound level of healing. This chapter turns its gaze toward the earth's bounty, unearthing the potent remedies cradled in its flora and the rhythmic movements that mimic the natural flow of life's currents. Here, amid the verdant expanses and beneath the canopy of the sky, lies the blueprint for mitigating the discomfort of joint pain and arthritis, conditions that tether many to the shores of discomfort and immobility.

11.1 NATURAL APPROACHES TO MANAGING JOINT PAIN AND ARTHRITIS

Anti-inflammatory diet for joint health

In the realm of dietary intervention, the adage "Let food be thy medicine" finds its most potent expression. An anti-inflammatory diet, rich in omega-3 fatty acids, antioxidants, and phytonutrients, operates much like a gentle tide, washing away the inflammation that often exacerbates joint pain. Cold-water fish such as salmon and mackerel, alongside a cornucopia of colorful fruits and vegetables, seeds like chia and flax, and spices known for their anti-inflammatory properties, including turmeric and ginger, compose the cornerstone of this dietary approach. The inclusion of whole grains and the eschewing of processed foods and sugars further augment this effort, fostering an internal environment where inflammation is quelled and pain finds little foothold.

Gentle exercise routines for mobility

The paradox of movement and arthritis is one that many find challenging; the very act of moving can incite discomfort, yet stagnation exacerbates the condition. Gentle exercise routines, calibrated to the rhythms of the body's capabilities, emerge as an elixir for enhancing flexibility and strengthening the muscles that support ailing joints. Tai Chi, with its fluid movements and emphasis on balance and deep breathing, mirrors the graceful flow of natural elements, offering a low-impact exercise alternative that soothes rather than strains. Similarly, water aerobics, performed in the supportive embrace of water, reduces the gravitational pull on painful joints, allowing for a range of motion that might otherwise be unattainable.

Supplements and herbs for joint support

Nature's apothecary, teeming with herbs and supplements, offers a constellation of remedies for those navigating the discomforts of arthritis. Curcumin, the active component in turmeric, stands out for its anti-inflammatory prowess, acting on biochemical pathways involved in inflammation. Omega-3 supplements, derived from fish oil or algae, contribute to this anti-inflammatory crusade, offering relief from the stiffness and pain that hallmark arthritis. Glucosamine and chondroitin, both naturally occurring substances within human cartilage, have been shown to aid in cushioning joints and supporting repair processes. These supplements, when integrated into a holistic health regimen, fortify the body's defenses against the ravages of arthritis.

Alternative therapies and treatments

Beyond the confines of conventional medicine, a spectrum of alternative therapies beckons, offering solace to those who tread the path of natural healing. Acupuncture, with its roots entwined in ancient Chinese medicine, employs the strategic insertion of needles to rebalance the body's energy flows, offering not just relief from pain but an enhanced sense of well-being. Massage therapy, through the skilled manipulation of the body's soft tissues, promotes circulation, eases muscle tension, and fosters a deep state of relaxation that can mitigate pain. The application of heat and cold, a remedy as old as time, provides immediate, though temporary, relief from joint pain, reducing inflammation and numbing the area to dull discomfort. These therapies, when chosen with care and incorporated into a comprehensive treatment plan, pave the way for improved joint function and a significant reduction in pain.

In navigating the multifaceted landscape of natural approaches to managing joint pain and arthritis, this chapter illuminates a path that intertwines the wisdom of the earth with the innate capacity of the body to heal and thrive. Through dietary adjustments, the gentle cadence of exercise, the strategic use of supplements, and the incorporation of alternative therapies, individuals find themselves empowered to reclaim their mobility and vitality. Here, in the embrace of nature's balm, lies the promise of a life unburdened by the constraints of pain, a life where movement is once again a source of joy rather than a reminder of limitations.

11.2 COGNITIVE HEALTH: PREVENTING MEMORY LOSS AND DEMENTIA

Brain-boosting foods and nutrients

In the verdant tapestry of cognitive well-being, the sustenance we derive from the earth plays a pivotal role, acting as both shield and elixir in the preservation of mental acuity. The nutrients that meander through our bloodstream, borne from the food we consume, hold sway over the intricate dance of neurons and synapses that underpin thought, memory, and cognition. Among these, omega-3 fatty acids, standing tall like sentinels, fortify the brain's structure, their presence in cell membranes enhancing fluidity and, thus, the efficiency of signal transmission. The venerable blueberry, with its deep hue mirroring the depths of the ocean, brings forth anthocyanins, potent antioxidants that quell the storm of oxidative stress, safeguarding neurons against the ravages of age. In their unassuming verdure, leafy greens carry a bounty of vitamins E and K, folate, and lutein, crafting a mosaic of protection that wards off cognitive decline. Walnuts, with their cerebral appearance, echo their affinity for brain health, delivering not just omega-3s but also polyphenolic compounds that stave off the harmful effects of inflammation and oxidative stress on neuronal pathways.

Mental exercises and activities

In its quest for eternal sharpness, the mind thrives not on rest but on the relentless pursuit of challenge and novelty. Much like a blacksmith's forge, cognitive training exercises temper the mind, enhancing its resilience against the encroachments of age. These exercises, ranging from puzzles that weave complex patterns of logic and reasoning to linguistic endeavors that stretch the boundaries of vocabulary and comprehension, ignite the synapses in a firework display of neural activity. Beyond the confines of structured exercises, hobbies that engage the mind in arts and crafts, music, and literature offer not just a respite from the mundane but a crucible for cognitive fortification. The act of learning a musical instrument, a language, or even the delicate strokes of painting etches new pathways in the brain, a testament to its boundless capacity for growth and adaptation.

The role of physical exercise in brain health

Amidst the myriad strategies for nurturing the mind, physical exercise emerges as a cornerstone, its benefits percolating through the blood-brain barrier to invigorate the very essence of cognitive function. Research delineates a clear trajectory from the rhythmic cadence of physical activity to the enhancement of memory, attention, and executive function. Aerobic exercise, in its myriad forms, catalyzes the release of neurotrophic factors, among which BDNF (brain-derived neurotrophic factor) reigns supreme, fostering the growth of new neurons and the fortification of synaptic connections. Resistance training, often overshadowed by its aerobic counterpart, stakes its claim in the cognitive realm, bolstering not just muscle but also the mind, enhancing spatial memory and executive function. This dual approach, marrying the vigor of aerobic activity with the resilience borne from resistance training, lays a foundation for cognitive health that withstands the test of time.

Sleep and cognitive function

In the tranquil embrace of sleep, the brain embarks on a nocturnal journey of consolidation and repair, a time when the experiences and learnings of the day are sifted, sorted, and embedded in the tapestry of memory. The sanctity of this process is underscored by the harmful effects of sleep disruption on cognitive function, where the erosion of memory, attention, and creative thought becomes palpably evident. The architecture of sleep, with its cycles of REM and non-REM stages, acts as the scaffold upon which memory consolidation is built, each phase playing its distinct role in the strengthening of neural connections and the purging of neural waste. Strategies for enhancing sleep quality and duration, therefore, become imperative in the preservation of cognitive health. Adherence to a sleep schedule that mirrors the body's natural circadian rhythms, the cultivation of pre-sleep rituals that signal the mind and body for rest, and the sanctification of the sleep environment as a haven from the intrusion of light and sound emerge as pillars supporting the edifice of cognitive well-being. In this realm, where sleep and cognition intertwine, the pursuit of restful slumber becomes not just an act of self-care but a bulwark against the tide of cognitive decline, safeguarding the clarity, creativity, and memory that define the essence of our humanity.

11.3 HEART HEALTH: COMBATING THE #1 KILLER WITH LIFESTYLE CHANGES

In the intricate dance of life, where vitality pulses through the very veins of our existence, the heart emerges not merely as a biological marvel but as the fulcrum around which the narrative of our health orbits. Amidst the cacophony of modern maladies, heart disease asserts its dominion, casting a shadow over the landscape of human wellness. Yet, within this shadow lies not despair but a call to action, a challenge to recalibrate our lifestyles in defiance of this silent adversary. Here, in the deliberate modulation of our daily habits, we find the keys to fortifying our heart against the encroachments of disease, transforming our routines into rituals of resilience.

Cardiovascular Benefits of a Plant-Based Diet

The alchemy of nutrition and heart health finds its most potent expression in the embrace of a plant-centric diet, a palette of verdant hues and earthy tones that paint a portrait of vitality and vigor. This dietary tapestry, woven from the fibers of fruits, vegetables, legumes, and grains, pulses with the life force of the natural world, offering not just sustenance but protection. Phytochemicals, those molecular artisans, work in the quiet sanctuaries of our bodies to mitigate inflammation, reduce oxidative stress, and lower the very biomarkers that herald heart disease. Fiber, in its humble abundance, escorts cholesterol from the body, while the complex symphony of vitamins and minerals orchestrates an environment where blood pressure is tempered and vessels remain supple. This plant-centric approach, far from a mere dietary preference, emerges as a profound act of rebellion against the tide of heart disease, a testament to the power of food as medicine.

Effective Exercise for Heart Health

The narrative of exercise and cardiovascular health unfolds like a grand epic, where each step, each stroke, each stretch contributes to the fortification of our heart's citadel. With their rhythmic cadence, aerobic activities emerge as the protagonists in this tale, and their efficacy in enhancing heart function and endurance is well documented. Running, cycling, and swimming, in their various expressions, invite the heart to beat with renewed strength, improving circulation and reducing the risk of heart disease. Yet, the plot thickens with the introduction of resistance training, a subplot that reveals the unexpected hero in the quest for heart health. By increasing lean muscle mass, we elevate our metabolic rate, a move that counteracts the specter of obesity and diabetes, both villains in the saga of cardiovascular disease. This balanced regimen, a harmonious blend of endurance and strength, composes a lifestyle where the heart's rhythm resonates with health and vitality.

Stress Management Techniques for Cardiovascular Well-Being

In the shadowed corners of our fast-paced existence, stress lurks as a silent saboteur of heart health, its insidious tendrils weaving through the fabric of our daily lives. The countermeasure to this pervasive threat lies not in the evasion of stress, an impossibility in our complex world, but in the mastery of its management. Techniques rooted in the ancient traditions of mindfulness and meditation offer a sanctuary from the storm, a place of calm amidst the chaos. Through focused breathing and the cultivation of present-moment awareness, we attenuate the body's stress response, a cascade of reactions that, left unchecked, erodes cardiovascular health. The practice of yoga, with its emphasis on breath control and postural alignment, serves as a bridge, connecting the mind's capacity for tranquility with the body's need for balance and flexibility. In these practices, we find not just a reprieve from stress but a blueprint for a heart-resilient lifestyle, where peace and calm preside over the storm of daily pressures.

Monitoring Heart Health Metrics

In the quest to shield our heart from the ravages of disease, knowledge emerges as our most formidable weapon. The metrics of heart health, indicators that whisper the secrets of our cardiovascular condition, beckon for our attention. Blood pressure, that vital sign of circulatory force, demands regular monitoring; its fluctuations are a map to understanding the terrain of our heart's health. Cholesterol levels, both LDL and HDL, serve as markers of lipid balance, guiding dietary and lifestyle adjustments. Blood sugar, often a silent herald of diabetes, requires vigilance, for its insidious rise portends trouble for the heart. When tracked with consistency, these metrics illuminate the path of our heart's journey through the landscape of health. Wearable technology, with its capacity for real-time monitoring and regular consultations with healthcare professionals, provides the tools and guidance necessary to navigate this path, ensuring that our heart beats to the rhythm of vitality and vigor.

In the narrative arc of heart health, where each choice and action contributes to the unfolding story of our well-being, the adoption of a plant-centric diet, an exercise regimen that balances endurance and strength, stress management techniques that anchor us in tranquility, and the vigilant monitoring of health metrics compose the chapters of a life lived in defiance of heart disease. Here, within the pages of this lifestyle manual, we script a tale of resilience, a testament to the power of intentional living in the cultivation of a heart that beats with the pulsing rhythm of health and longevity.

11.4 DIABETES PREVENTION AND MANAGEMENT THROUGH LIFESTYLE

In the intricate dance with our biology, the specter of diabetes looms, a testament to the era's excesses and sedentary inclinations. Yet, within this challenge lies an opportunity—a call to recalibrate our lifestyles in harmony with the rhythms of health that pulse through the natural world. The modulation of our habits, from the food that fuels our existence to the vigor of our movements and the tranquility of our minds, emerges as a potent antidote to the insidious creep of this malady.

The alchemy of lifestyle modification begins in the crucible of our daily sustenance. A nuanced understanding of the triad of macronutrients—carbohydrates, fats, and proteins—becomes essential. The quality and quantity of carbohydrates consumed profoundly influence blood sugar levels. Whole grains, legumes, and vegetables, rich in fiber, ensure a moderated release of glucose into the bloodstream, preventing the abrupt spikes that challenge insulin's regulatory capacity. Fats, particularly those of the unsaturated kind found in nuts, seeds, and avocados, contribute not just to satiety but to maintaining cell membrane integrity and hormonal balance, factors critical in insulin sensitivity. Proteins, with their minimal impact on blood glucose, serve as the bedrock for muscle and tissue repair, stabilizing blood sugar levels indirectly by enhancing metabolic function.

The narrative of dietary management is incomplete without addressing the symphony of micronutrients—vitamins, minerals, and phytochemicals—that play supportive roles in this metabolic ballet. Magnesium, found in leafy greens and whole grains, and chromium, present in broccoli and potatoes, assist in fine-tuning glucose metabolism and insulin sensitivity. Incorporating these elements into a cohesive dietary strategy does not merely aim at managing diabetes but at rekindling the body's innate capacity for balance and self-regulation.

Parallel to the dietary strategy runs the vital current of physical activity. Exercise, in its myriad forms, acts directly upon the canvas of our physiology, enhancing the uptake of glucose into muscle cells and igniting the metabolic pathways that improve insulin sensitivity. The spectrum of beneficial physical activities spans from the brisk rhythm of walking to the structured challenges of resistance training, each modality contributing its unique brush-strokes to the masterpiece of metabolic health. Beyond its immediate effects on glucose control, exercise weaves resilience into the fabric of our being, fortifying the heart, invigorating the mind, and sculpting the body's contours in defiance of diabetes' advance.

Amidst the physical transformations wrought by diet and exercise, the subtler realm of stress management beckons for attention. The turbulence of stress, with its cascade of hormonal upheavals, disrupts the delicate balance of glucose in the blood, nudging the body towards insulin resistance. The cultivation of tranquility, therefore, becomes not merely a pursuit of mental serenity but a strategic intervention in the metabolic symphony. Techniques that anchor awareness in the present moment, from the deliberate breaths of mindfulness meditation to the gentle postures of yoga, dissipate the storm clouds of stress, restoring calm to the body's internal environment. This calm, in turn, stabilizes blood sugar levels, closing the loop in the holistic management of diabetes.

As we navigate the complexities of preventing and managing diabetes through lifestyle changes, the principles of balance, moderation, and mindfulness emerge as guiding stars. The integration of dietary wisdom, the discipline of physical activity, and the serenity of stress management into the tapestry of daily life does not merely ward off the specter of diabetes but elevates our existence to a higher plane of vitality and harmony. In this elevated state, we find not just health but a profound connection to the cycles and rhythms of the natural world, a reminder that, in the end, our well-being is deeply intertwined with the health of the planet that sustains us.

In closing, this chapter's essence encapsulates the transformative power of lifestyle changes in diabetes prevention and management. It underscores the significance of dietary mindfulness, the vitality imbued by physical activity, and the equilibrium fostered through stress management as pillars supporting the edifice of health. As we turn our gaze forward, let this understanding serve as a beacon, guiding us toward a future where well-being is nurtured as a holistic endeavor grounded in the wisdom of our bodies and the healing embrace of the natural world.

EMBRACING THE HORIZON: THE VANGUARD OF LONGEVITY SCIENCE

At the confluence of tradition and innovation, where the ancient rhythms of nature meet the precision of modern science, a new frontier in the quest for longevity and wellness emerges. This terrain, uncharted yet pulsing with potential, invites a closer examination of the mechanisms that govern aging, offering glimpses into a future where the boundaries of life itself may be extended through scientific discovery. The pursuit of longevity, once the domain of philosophers and alchemists, now finds its champions among geneticists, biotechnologists, and pioneers in the field of regenerative medicine, each contributing to a mosaic of knowledge that could redefine human healthspan.

Cutting-edge research in Longevity and Anti-Aging

In laboratories and research institutions around the globe, a revolution unfolds, propelled by the quest to decipher the molecular narratives of aging. Recent breakthroughs in longevity science spotlight the malleability of our biological clocks, suggesting that the rate at which we age may be more within our control than previously imagined. Among these discoveries, the role of telomeres and the enzyme telomerase in cellular aging stands out, offering clues to how we might one day reverse the tide of biological decline. Advances in genetic editing technologies, particularly CRISPR-Cas9, herald a new era where genetic predispositions to age-related diseases could be altered, paving the way for personalized therapies that extend healthspan with precision and efficacy.

Genetics and Longevity

The labyrinth of human genetics, with its complex interplay of genes and environment, holds secrets to longevity that researchers are only beginning to understand. Insights into the genetic profiles of centenarians, individuals who have crossed the threshold of 100 years, reveal patterns and mutations that confer resistance to age-related illnesses. These findings, while still in their infancy, suggest that future treatments could mimic these genetic advantages, offering a blueprint for extending life. Integrating big data analytics into longevity research further accelerates this exploration, enabling scientists to sift through vast datasets to identify genetic markers associated with healthy aging, a process akin to finding needles in a haystack but with the potential to uncover the genetic foundations of a long, healthy life.

Emerging Technologies in Health Monitoring

In the quest for longevity, knowledge is power, and the power to know comes from the data collected about our bodies. Wearable technologies and digital health tools represent a significant leap forward in this arena, transforming everyday objects into sentinels of health. Smartwatches that monitor heart rate, sleep patterns, and even blood oxygen levels provide a continuous stream of data, offering insights into the rhythms and fluctuations of our bodies.

These devices, once the purview of athletes and fitness enthusiasts, now beckon to anyone with an interest in personal health, promising a granular view of our biological status in real-time. The proliferation of these technologies democratizes health monitoring, putting the tools for longevity in the hands of the many rather than the few.

The Potential of Regenerative Medicine

At the vanguard of longevity science lies regenerative medicine, a field that seeks not just to halt or slow aging but to reverse its effects, restoring vitality and function to tissues and organs. Stem cell therapy, with its ability to repair damaged cells and regenerate lost tissues, stands at the forefront of this movement. Already, treatments derived from stem cells offer hope for conditions ranging from heart disease to macular degeneration, hinting at a future where the decline of age can be countered with the renewal of life at a cellular level. Tissue engineering, another pillar of regenerative medicine, combines scaffolds, cells, and biologically active molecules to reconstruct or replace damaged organs, offering the promise of a future where organ failure is not an inevitability of aging but a challenge to overcome.

This chapter, a tapestry woven from the threads of cutting-edge research and emerging technologies, paints a picture of a future where the boundaries of aging are not fixed but fluid, subject to the ebb and flow of scientific discovery. It is a future where the pursuit of longevity transcends the quest for mere survival, aspiring instead to a life marked by vitality, resilience, and an enduring zest for the wonders that each new day holds.

12.2 THE NEXT GENERATION OF BIOHACKS: WHAT'S ON THE HORIZON

In the ever-evolving tableau of human health and longevity, the concept of biohacking emerges as a beacon for those seeking to fine-tune the delicate machinery of their biology. This pursuit, grounded in the desire to transcend the limitations traditionally imposed by our genetic blueprint and environmental circumstances, enters a new epoch marked by innovations that promise to redefine the boundaries of what it means to live a healthy, extended life. The horizon glows with the nascent light of biohacking trends, synthetic biology, neurohacking, and the dawn of personalized nutrition, each heralding a future where the alchemy of science and nature coalesces into unprecedented modalities for wellness enhancement.

Innovative Biohacking Trends

The landscape of biohacking is fertile, teeming with burgeoning techniques poised to transition from the fringes to the mainstream. Among these, the manipulation of the body's microbiome stands as a testament to the intricate relationship between human health and the trillions of microorganisms that inhabit our bodies. Emerging research underscores the potential to modulate this microbial ecosystem through targeted probiotic strains, prebiotic fibers, and even fecal microbiota transplants, aiming to restore balance and forestall disease. Concurrently, the exploration of chronobiology, the science of biological rhythms, offers a panoramic view of how syncing our lifestyle with our circadian rhythms—be it through controlled light exposure, meal timing, or sleep scheduling—can amplify metabolic efficiency, cognitive function, and overall well-being. These trends, rooted in a deeper understanding of our biological underpinnings, signal a shift towards biohacking practices that harmonize with the body's natural tendencies, promising a future where health optimization is both nuanced and deeply personalized.

Synthetic Biology and Its Implications for Health

On the cusp of this new era, synthetic biology emerges, blurring the lines between biology and engineering, promising to recalibrate our approach to health and disease. This discipline, characterized by the design and fabrication of biological components and systems not found in the natural world, holds the promise of creating bespoke solutions to aging and illness. Imagine cells engineered to seek out and dismantle cancerous growths, bacteria reprogrammed to produce essential nutrients at optimal levels, or even the development of synthetic organs tailor-made to replace their failing biological counterparts. The implications of synthetic biology for health and longevity are profound, offering a vision of the future where each individual's biological needs are met with precision-crafted solutions, rendering diseases that currently elude cure manageable, if not entirely obsolete.

Neurohacking for Cognitive Enhancement

As the frontier of biohacking expands, so too does the realm of possibilities for enhancing one of our most precious assets: our cognitive capabilities. Neurohacking, a term that encapsulates various techniques aimed at optimizing brain function, stands at the vanguard of this movement. Advances in non-invasive brain stimulation technologies, such as transcranial direct current stimulation (tDCS) and transcranial magnetic stimulation (TMS), offer tantalizing glimpses into methods for enhancing learning, memory, and creativity without the scalpel or pharmacological side effects. Coupled with the burgeoning field of nootropics, substances ranging from well-known compounds like caffeine to novel peptides and smart drugs, neurohacking presages a future where mental acuity, focus, and resilience against neurodegenerative diseases are within our grasp, customizable and accessible.

The Future of Personalized Nutrition

Amidst the constellation of innovations in the biohacking universe, personalized nutrition shines brightly, heralding a departure from one-size-fits-all dietary recommendations to a future where food is medicine tailored to the individual's unique genetic makeup, lifestyle and health goals. This vision is propelled by advances in genomics, metabolomics, and artificial intelligence, converging to analyze the complex interplay between nutrients and our biology. The potential for machine learning algorithms to sift through this data, identifying patterns and making predictions about how specific dietary components influence gene expression, inflammation, and metabolic pathways, is groundbreaking. In the future, a simple saliva test could yield dietary guidelines crafted to optimize one's health, mitigate predispositions to diseases, and even slow the aging process. Personalized nutrition, in this light, becomes not just a tool for disease prevention but a daily practice of health cultivation grounded in the specificity of our biological individuality.

In the tapestry of future biohacking trends, each thread - from the burgeoning practices set to enter the mainstream, through the revolutionary potential of synthetic biology and neurohacking, to the dawn of truly personalized nutrition - interweaves to form a picture of a future where longevity is not left to chance but cultivated with intention and scientific precision. This horizon, vibrant with the promise of innovation, invites us to reimagine the boundaries of health and wellness, heralding an era where the full potential of human vitality can be realized.

12.3 THE ROLE OF PERSONALIZED MEDICINE IN WELLNESS

In an era marked by rapid advancements in science and technology, the healthcare domain stands on the brink of a paradigmatic shift with the advent of personalized medicine. This emergent discipline, marrying the intricacies of one's genetic makeup with the nuances of their lifestyle and environmental contexts, heralds a new dawn in preventive and therapeutic healthcare. Far removed from the traditional one-size-fits-all approach, personalized medicine navigates the unique biochemical pathways etched into an individual's being, crafting interventions and treatments with unparalleled precision.

At the heart of this transformation lies the profound potential to recalibrate disease prevention and management strategies. By illuminating the genetic predispositions harbored within the depths of one's DNA, personalized medicine offers a preemptive strike against the specter of hereditary diseases, shifting the narrative from reaction to prevention. This approach, nuanced and deeply informed by data, ensures that therapeutic interventions are not merely general but genetically attuned, drastically improving their efficacy. In conditions ranging from the complexities of cancer to the metabolic pathways influenced in diabetes, treatments tailored to the individual's genetic profile promise a significant leap in medical outcomes.

Integrating personalized medicine into daily health routines emerges not as a distant future but as an accessible present. The advent of genetic testing and personalized health assessments, once confined to specialized medical facilities, now reaches into the homes and lives of individuals, offering insights into the genetic blueprints that predispose them to certain conditions. This democratization of genetic information empowers individuals to make informed decisions about their health, lifestyle adjustments, and preventative measures, fostering a proactive stance towards wellness. With a simple saliva sample, one can unravel the mysteries of their genetic inheritance, paving the way for a life not just lived but optimized.

Yet, as we tread this promising path, ethical and privacy considerations cast a long shadow. The sanctity of one's genetic data, a diary of their biological inheritance, demands rigorous safeguards against breaches of privacy and misuse. The potential for genetic information to influence employment, insurance, and even social standing raises pertinent questions about discrimination and consent. Navigating this landscape requires a delicate balance, ensuring that the benefits of personalized medicine do not come at the cost of one's right to privacy and autonomy. Regulatory frameworks and ethical guidelines, evolving in tandem with these advancements, strive to protect individuals, ensuring that the journey toward personalized wellness remains both safe and just.

In this landscape, where the confluence of genetics, lifestyle, and environment shapes the trajectory of one's health, personalized medicine emerges as a beacon of hope. It promises a future where health is not merely managed but optimized, where therapies are not just applied but crafted, and where the nuances of individuality are not overlooked but celebrated. This vision of healthcare, deeply personal and intricately tailored, stands as a testament to the potential inherent in the marriage of technology and human ingenuity, guiding us towards a horizon where wellness is both a personal journey and a collective achievement.

12.4 STAYING AHEAD: CONTINUOUS LEARNING FOR LIFELONG HEALTH

In a world awash with information, pursuing health literacy becomes not merely a choice but a necessity for those aiming to navigate the complexities of wellness with understanding and insight. The crux of this endeavor lies in recognizing that the landscape of health knowledge is not static but dynamically evolving, shaped by the relentless march of scientific discovery and the ever-changing tapestry of societal norms. Thus, the commitment to staying informed and sieving through the burgeoning expanse of health-related data emerges as a foundational pillar for those aspiring to optimize their well-being.

With the proliferation of digital platforms, the avenues for expanding one's health knowledge have multiplied, offering access to a wealth of resources that span the spectrum from the elemental to the esoteric. Books, meticulously penned by pioneers in the fields of medicine, nutrition, and psychology, serve as beacons, illuminating the nuanced pathways through which health can be nurtured and sustained. Online courses, ranging from informal webinars to structured programs offered by leading universities, provide a scaffold for understanding, allowing individuals to delve deep into specific areas of interest, from the molecular underpinnings of aging to the holistic principles of Eastern medicine.

Websites and blogs, curated by experts and enthusiasts alike, offer a mosaic of perspectives, each contributing to a broader understanding of what it means to live well. Podcasts, marrying the intimacy of voice with the convenience of digital access, bring the insights of health professionals, researchers, and thought leaders directly to the listener, transforming commutes and leisurely walks into opportunities for learning. The selection of these resources, guided by discernment and a critical eye, ensures that the information absorbed is not only current but credible, a distillation of wisdom that can be integrated into the fabric of one's daily life.

Yet, the quest for health literacy extends beyond the solitary act of consumption, flourishing in the rich soil of community engagement. Forums, workshops, and seminars, whether virtual or in physical spaces, foster an environment of shared inquiry where questions are posed, debates are kindled, and experiences are exchanged. This collective journey into knowledge, underscored by the diversity of its participants, enriches the learning experience, embedding it with a multitude of perspectives that challenge and refine one's understanding. It is within these communal gatherings that the abstract becomes tangible, as theories are woven into the fabric of real-life stories, bridging the gap between knowledge and application.

The dynamism of health information, with its constant flux and flow, necessitates a strategy for assimilating new insights while reassessing established beliefs. This process, iterative and reflective, involves scrutinizing the source and integrity of new findings and juxtaposing them against the bedrock of one's existing knowledge. It demands an openness to revision, a willingness to recalibrate one's practices in light of fresh evidence or innovative methodologies. The integration of new health information, therefore, becomes an exercise in adaptability, a dance between the known and the unknown, guided by the principles of critical thinking and evidence-based decision-making.

In this fluid interplay of learning and unlearning, the individual emerges not as a passive recipient of information but as an active participant in co-creating their health narrative. The resources at their disposal, from the written word to the shared wisdom of communities, serve as tools and allies in this endeavor. They empower the individual to sculpt a lifestyle that is not just reactive to the ailments of the day but proactive in the cultivation of vitality and resilience.

As we draw the curtains on this exploration of continuous learning and its pivotal role in fostering lifelong health, we are reminded of the broader vista that unfolds before us. This commitment to health literacy, the relentless pursuit of knowledge, and the adaptive integration of new insights into our lives stand as a testament to our capacity for growth and transformation. It reaffirms the belief that the journey toward optimal well-being is not a solitary endeavor but a collective voyage enriched by the contributions of science, tradition, and community. In this journey, each step forward, informed by learning and shaped by the wisdom of shared experiences, brings us closer to realizing the full potential of our health and vitality.

CONCLUSION

As we draw this journey of discovery to a close, I reflect on the intricate tapestry we've explored together—a journey through the realms of longevity and wellness, where the fusion of cutting-edge biohacks and the wisdom of age-old practices has illuminated our path. The integration of red-light therapy, grounding, and hydrogen water, alongside the invaluable insights of Gary Brecka, has marked pivotal milestones in our quest for a vibrant, enduring life. These elements, each a thread in the broader weave of health, underscore the holistic approach necessary for aging not just with grace but with vitality.

The narrative of this book has been deeply personal, rooted in my own health challenges and the profound impact of my wife's illness on our collective wellness journey. It's a testament to the universal desire for health and longevity that knows no bounds, touching each of us with the promise of a fuller, more vibrant life. This shared aspiration binds us, encouraging a reflection on the indelible link between our physical and mental well-being.

We've delved into the essential strategies for aging gracefully—managing inflammation through mindful diet choices, unlocking the rejuvenating power of autophagy, reaping the benefits of intermittent fasting, and embracing physical activity tailored to our unique stages of life. Each strategy, presented with both depth and accessibility, is designed to equip you with the knowledge and tools necessary for embarking on this transformative journey.

Yet, knowledge without action is like a seed unplanted. The insights and information within these pages serve as a blueprint for practical, actionable steps you can integrate into your daily life, offering both immediate and enduring benefits to your health and well-being. It's a call to action—a pledge to yourself to take charge of your health journey, regardless of the starting point.

As we navigate the ever-evolving landscape of longevity and wellness, the value of continuous learning and adaptation cannot be overstated. Please remain voraciously curious and open to the wealth of new research and developments that promise to further our understanding and capabilities in this field.

In making a personal commitment to your health, remember the power of community. Engaging with like-minded individuals offers a wellspring of support, motivation, and shared wisdom that can amplify your efforts and enrich your journey. Whether through local groups, online forums, or wellness programs, connecting with others can transform the solitary pursuit of health into a shared voyage of discovery and growth.

In closing, I extend to you a message of hope and empowerment. Don't let your journey of wellness and longevity be rooted in a life-changing event for you or the ones you love. Don't let the pursuit of your career or anything else distract you from your health and wellness, as it did me. The journey toward optimal health and longevity is within your grasp; each step forward is a testament to your resilience, your capacity for change, and your unwavering commitment to living your fullest life. Embrace this journey with optimism, patience, and perseverance, and know that each small change can beget monumental shifts in your well-being.

In health and hope,

Max

REFERENCES

- *Epigenetics and lifestyle - PMC* https://www.ncbi.nlm.nih.gov/pmc/articles/PMC3752894/
- *Telomere extension turns back aging clock in cultured human ...* https://med.stanford.edu/news/all-news/2015/01/telomere-extension-turns-back-aging-clock-in-cultured-cells.html
- *Inflammation Discovery Could Slow Aging, Prevent Age-Related Diseases* https://newsroom.uvahealth.com/2023/07/24/inflammation-discovery-could-slow-aging-prevent-age-related-diseases/
- *Autophagy Fasting: What You Should Know Before Starting ...* https://www.insidetracker.com/a/articles/autophagy-fasting-what-you-should-know-before-starting#:~:
- *Developing a Growth Mindset Can Make Aging Easier* https://medium.com/crows-feet/developing-a-growth-mindset-can-make-aging-easier-d2cddfe2ef41
- *Association Between Subjective Well-being and Living Longer ...* https://www.ncbi.nlm.nih.gov/pmc/articles/PMC6624816/#:~:
- *Mental health of older adults* https://www.who.int/news-room/fact-sheets/detail/mental-health-of-older-adults
- *Ways of Bolstering Resilience in Older Adults* https://melissainstitute.org/wp-content/uploads/2016/09/Ways-of-bolstering-resilience-in-older-adults.pdf
- *Healthy Longevity | The Nutrition Source - hsph.harvard.edu* https://www.hsph.harvard.edu/nutritionsource/healthy-longevity/
- *Nutritional Profile and Potential Health Benefits of Super ...* https://www.mdpi.com/2071-1050/13/16/9240
- *Summary of Bio Hacking Will Save Your Life - Gary Brecka* https://www.summarize.tech/www.youtube.com/watch?v=V0ujXACQNd4#:~:
- *Fasting, circadian rhythms, and time restricted feeding in ...* https://www.ncbi.nlm.nih.gov/pmc/articles/PMC5388543/
- *Growing Stronger - Strength Training for Older Adults* https://www.cdc.gov/physicalactivity/downloads/growing_stronger.pdf
- *Cycling or swimming, walking or yoga: What is the best exercise for you?* https://www.irishtimes.com/life-and-style/health-family/fitness/cycling-or-swimming-walking-or-yoga-what-is-the-best-exercise-for-you-1.4139394

- *Taking balance training for older adults one step further* https://www.ncbi.nlm.nih.gov/pmc/articles/PMC4419050/
- *GARY BRECKA: HUMAN BIOLOGIST & BIO HACKER | THE ...* https://www.garybrecka.com/
- *Summary of Bio Hacking Will Save Your Life - Gary Brecka* https://www.summarize.tech/www.youtube.com/watch?v=V0ujXACQNd4#:~:
- *NASA Research Illuminates Medical Uses of Light* https://spinoff.nasa.gov/NASA-Research-Illuminates-Medical-Uses-of-Light
- *Cold temperature extends longevity and prevents disease ...* https://www.nature.com/articles/s43587-023-00383-4
- *Grounding – The universal anti-inflammatory remedy - PMC* https://www.ncbi.nlm.nih.gov/pmc/articles/PMC10105021/
- *Food Secrets of the World's Longest-Lived People* https://www.bluezones.com/2020/07/blue-zones-diet-food-secrets-of-the-worlds-longest-lived-people/
- *Moai—This Tradition is Why Okinawan People Live Longer ...* https://www.bluezones.com/2018/08/moai-this-tradition-is-why-okinawan-people-live-longer-better/
- *13 Unusual Ways to Shed Stress (Lessons ... - Blue Zones* https://www.bluezones.com/2022/02/13-unusual-ways-to-shed-stress-lessons-from-the-worlds-blue-zones/
- *Physical Activity in Centenarians beyond Cut-Point-Based ...* https://www.ncbi.nlm.nih.gov/pmc/articles/PMC9517573/
- *Can meditation slow rate of cellular aging? Cognitive ...* https://www.ncbi.nlm.nih.gov/pmc/articles/PMC3057175/
- *Strong evidence that yoga protects against frailty in older adults* https://news.harvard.edu/gazette/story/2023/03/strong-evidence-that-yoga-protects-against-frailty-in-older-adults/
- *GARY BRECKA: HUMAN BIOLOGIST & BIO HACKER | THE ...* https://www.garybrecka.com/
- *Effect of breathwork on stress and mental health: A meta- ...* https://www.nature.com/articles/s41598-022-27247-y
- *Summary of Bio Hacking Will Save Your Life - Gary Brecka* https://www.summarize.tech/www.youtube.com/watch?v=V0ujXACQNd4#:~
- *Study Probes Connection Between Excessive Screen Media ...* https://medicine.yale.edu/news-article/yale-study-probes-connection-between-excessive-screen-media-activity-and-mental-health-problems-in-youth/
- *5 Ways to Reduce Toxic Exposures in Your Home* https://www.ewg.org/news-insights/news/5-ways-reduce-toxic-exposures-your-home

- *Red Light and the Sleep Quality and Endurance ...* https://www.ncbi.nlm.nih.gov/pmc/articles/PMC3499892/
- *Summary of Bio Hacking Will Save Your Life - Gary Brecka* https://www.summarize.tech/www.youtube.com/watch?v=V0ujXACQNd4#:~:
- *A Controlled Trial to Determine the Efficacy of Red and Near-Infrared Light Treatment in Patient Satisfaction, Reduction of Fine Lines, Wrinkles, Skin Roughness, and Intradermal Collagen Density Increase* https://www.ncbi.nlm.nih.gov/pmc/articles/PMC3926176/
- *Be SMART about setting health-related goals | Diet and Nutrition* https://utswmed.org/medblog/smart-goals-health-wellness/
- *The Best Fitness Trackers for 2024* https://www.pcmag.com/picks/the-best-fitness-trackers
- *How Does Social Connectedness Affect Health?* https://www.cdc.gov/emotional-wellbeing/social-connectedness/affect-health.htm
- *Summary of Bio Hacking Will Save Your Life - Gary Brecka* https://www.summarize.tech/www.youtube.com/watch?v=V0ujXACQNd4#:~:
- *Effects of Group Fitness Classes on Stress and Quality ...* https://pubmed.ncbi.nlm.nih.gov/29084328/
- *Volunteering and its Surprising Benefits* https://www.helpguide.org/articles/healthy-living/volunteering-and-its-surprising-benefits.htm
- *Summary of Bio Hacking Will Save Your Life - Gary Brecka* https://www.summarize.tech/www.youtube.com/watch?v=V0ujXACQNd4#:~:
- *A Controlled Trial to Determine the Efficacy of Red and Near-Infrared Light Treatment in Patient Satisfaction, Reduction of Fine Lines, Wrinkles, Skin Roughness, and Intradermal Collagen Density Increase* https://www.ncbi.nlm.nih.gov/pmc/articles/PMC3926176/
- *Stress relief tips for older adults* https://www.health.harvard.edu/stress/stress-relief-tips-for-older-adults
- *Plant Based Diet and Its Effect on Cardiovascular Disease* https://www.ncbi.nlm.nih.gov/pmc/articles/PMC9963093/#:~:
- *Summary of Bio Hacking Will Save Your Life - Gary Brecka* https://www.summarize.tech/www.youtube.com/watch?v=V0ujXACQNd4#:~:
- *2023 Breakthroughs in longevity research - Timeline* https://www.timeline.com/blog/breakthroughs-in-healthy-aging-2023-top-health-span-research#:~:*Reverse skin aging signs by red light photobiomodulation* https://www.ncbi.nlm.nih.gov/pmc/articles/PMC10311288/
- *Advances in Regenerative Medicine and Tissue Engineering* https://www.ncbi.nlm.nih.gov/pmc/articles/PMC6091336/